NCLEX-RN 2020-2021

New Outline + Study Guide with 400 Test Questions and Detailed Answer Explanations (Includes 4 Full Practice Exams and Nursing Certification Review)

Table of Contents

Introduction

Nursing is both an art and a science. As an art, the nursing practice attends to the social and emotional needs of patients. This practice requires sensitivity, compassion and emotional intelligence, skills that can't be assessed by objective methods. As a science, the nursing practice is built on the objective principles of biological, psychological, physical and social sciences.

The nursing practice is continuously evolving in its approach to patient care. As a discipline, it harnesses the principles of critical thinking to integrate science, technology and nursing care.

The Purpose of a Registered Nurse

Currently, there are about 2.86 million registered nurses in the United States, with an average nurse-to-doctor ratio of 3:1. Nurses have the most direct contact with clients. Thus, registered nurses are key figures in the health-care sector. Apart from providing personalized care to clients, they are important contributors to the efficient delivery of health-care services. Services which nurses provide include:

Nursing Care – Registered nurses provide expert, personalized care to clients. Such care includes evaluating clients' symptoms, monitoring vital signs and administering drugs. They also assist clients with eating, bed positioning, bathing, walking and performing daily activities. Nursing care also includes providing emotional support in the form of therapeutic communication and social interaction.

Health Administration – Registered nurses record and maintain their clients' health information. They are actively involved in the delegation, supervision and prioritization of nursing care. For example, registered nurses supervise and delegate tasks to nursing assistants and licensed practical nurses (LPNs). To do this, a registered nurse has to teach, mentor and assess the strengths and weaknesses of individual nursing assistants and LPNs. This task requires the use of efficient teaching skills, communication and leadership.

Nurses regularly collaborate with other medical professionals. For example, nurses provide valuable information to doctors on their clients' progress, emotional states, social and emotional challenges. A registered nurse collaborates with hysiotherapists, radiographers, psychologists, dietitians, specialist nurse practitioners and other health-care workers in health-care settings. Furthermore, registered nurses often engage in policy-making and administration that affect the way health services are provided to the public.

Health Education – Registered nurses are professional health educators. Whether it's educating clients or LPNs and nursing assistants, they provide expert care on health safety, primary, secondary and tertiary prevention methods. For this reason, registered nurses not only work in health facilities but in schools, industries, home centers and just about any environment where health and safety is required.

Who is a Registered Nurse?

A registered nurse holds a nursing diploma, an associate degree in nursing, a bachelor of science in nursing and has passed the NCLEX-RN exam administered by the National Council of State Boards of Nursing (NCSBN).

Diploma Programs

Nursing diploma programs are hospital-based programs that offer hands-on practical knowledge alongside theoretical information. Training usually lasts for one to three years. As diploma programs were the first form of training available for nurses, it is no wonder that there are more nurses with nursing diplomas than other nursing degrees. However, the popularity of nursing diplomas has declined in recent years because employers now require a minimum of a two-year associate degree in nursing.

Associate Degree Programs

This is the most common route of nursing education for students. The degree is less expensive when compared to a bachelor's degree, and education is more comprehensive than a diploma. Students are trained in the theories of basic medical science, clinical medicine, social science, nursing theory and nursing practice. Also, hands-on training is provided in health settings. It takes about two years to complete an associate degree program in nursing.

Baccalaureate Programs

About a decade ago, the nursing profession unanimously decided to make baccalaureate programs the profession's preferred program of choice. To do this, they created an ambitious goal to have at least 80% of practicing registered nurses (RNs) obtain a bachelor's degree in nursing science by 2020. They were successful in meeting that goal.

These days, the entry-level requirement for most health organizations is the bachelor of science in nursing (BSN). Some organizations have higher remuneration for nurses with a BSN. A bachelor's degree also provides more opportunities for career promotion into nursing specialties, nursing management and administrative positions. A BSN is the minimum requirement for a master's or doctoral degree in nursing.

Although an associate degree in nursing is the minimum educational requirement for a registered nurse, the medical community encourages RNs to seek a BSN, even after getting a diploma or an associate degree. The idea is to encourage continued learning in the nursing profession. To make this possible, nursing schools offer flexible pathways for students to earn a BSN. One way is to offer post-licensure programs to RNs with a diploma or an associate degree in nursing. Such programs last one to two years. Some organizations also offer 12-18-month BSN pre-licensure programs for people with college degrees who wish to become registered nurses.

Traditional BSN Program

A traditional BSN takes four years to complete. The coursework is in-depth, offering comprehensive information on nursing theory, practice, humanities, social sciences and nursing research.

Accelerated BSN Programs

Accelerated BSN programs are ideal for college graduates who want to pursue a career in nursing. These programs take about two years to complete. These programs are intense and demanding, with a modified curriculum that shortens the usual time for clinical education. The programs include coursework in the summer, with no breaks in between semesters.

RN to BSN Completion Programs

These programs are available for nursing graduates without a BSN degree. Graduates with a nursing diploma or associate degree do not have to go back to college for a four-year BSN program. Instead, they can do a two-year RN to BSN program to fast-track the process. Most of these programs are flexible, offering part-time, online and assistance programs for nurses.

Career Options

A registered nurse has a wide range of career options, not limited to health facilities.

Career Options in Hospital Settings

Registered nurses can work as general hospital nurses or in specialties like midwifery, psychiatry, pediatrics, oncology, urology and trauma. Registered nurses can go a step further to become advanced practice registered nurses.

These nurses have in-depth and specialized knowledge and are licensed to provide advanced professional care to clients. Some examples include nurse midwives, nurse practitioners, certified registered nurse anesthetists and clinical nurse specialists.

Career Options Outside of Hospital Settings

Registered nurses can also work outside of hospital settings as school nurses, flight nurses, travel nurses, nurse educators, home health nurses, nursing informatics technicians, forensic nurses and public health nurses.

Remuneration

The salary of a registered nurse averages $75,510 per year, and about $36.30 per hour. Factors that affect remuneration include level of education, type of nursing degree, experience, location and employer. All in all, a newly licensed RN should earn between $45,000-$60,000 per year.

Pros and Cons of Becoming a Registered Nurse

It's good to evaluate the pros and cons of choosing to become a registered nurse before following that career path.

Pros

Humanitarian Service – Like other health-related services, nurses provide direct service to humans. It can be deeply rewarding to use your skills, time and expertise to save a life.

Growth – Although most nurses prefer to advance their careers in a hospital setting, there are lots of opportunities for growth elsewhere.

Flexible Schedules – Nurses can work full-time, part-time or on an on-call basis. Calls typically include 12-hour work shifts with off-call days.

Job Security – There will always be a demand for health-care services because people always need medical care. Like other health-related careers, nursing is lucrative, with few layoffs and little unemployment.

Adventure – A nursing career is an adventurous one. Nurses come in contact with different clients who have unique needs. And it is always exciting to see clients recover from their illnesses.

Cons

Long Hours – Nurses work long hours that may include 12-hour shifts, night shifts and call duties. Nurses work every day of the week, all year round, on weekends and during summer holidays and public holidays.

Emotional and Physical Burnout – Like other health workers, nurses are vulnerable to emotional and physical burnout. This is because providing care to sick people is demanding. Nursing involves a lot of physical activity, including carrying, lifting and pushing. Also, nurses provide emotional support and compassion to all their clients. Nurses have to deal with the loss of their clients, even after putting in maximum effort to save their lives. Nurses have to make split-second decisions in critical cases and emergencies.

Exposure to Biohazards – Nurses are vulnerable to biohazards like needle-prick injuries, infected aerosols, infected contact surfaces and radiation. Biohazards can be life-threatening. Sometimes, they may be difficult to prevent.

Psychological Hazards – Nurses are vulnerable to psychological hazards that can come in the form of verbal and physical violence from clients and their relatives. Nurses are at an even greater risk of experiencing violence. The US Department of Labor states that 45% of health-care workplace violence is directed against nurses. Violence can not only come from clients and their relatives but also from superiors.

Chapter 1: The NCLEX-RN Exam

What is the NCLEX-RN?

After obtaining a nursing degree, a graduate will need a license from the appropriate licensing body. Nurses are required to take a licensing exam offered by the National Council of State Boards of Nursing. This licensing exam is the National Council Licensure Examination for Registered Nurses (NCLEX-RN).

The NCLEX-RN exam tests the skills and knowledge of entry-level nurses. The aim of the exam is simple: to determine whether a nurse is safe enough to be licensed for practice. The test questions are administered by the NCSBN, on behalf of the member boards. These member boards include nursing boards in the 10 provinces in Canada, the 50 states in the US, the district of Columbia and the four US territories, which are American Samoa, the Northern Mariana Islands, Guam and the US Virgin Islands.

NCLEX exams are given in a computer-adaptive testing format, supervised by the Pearson Professional Centers. In these computerized exams, the software algorithm selects questions from a question bank. Selection is based on how well a candidate answers the previous question. The NCLEX-RN has a wide range of questions in its question bank, designed to test examinees' ability to think critically.

The NCSBN prides itself on its meticulous development of the NCLEX test plan. The structure of the exams is tailored after Bloom's taxonomy for the cognitive domain, a higher level of cognitive ability that uses complex thought processing and critical thinking.

Before new tests are created, the board conducts research on the current practice of an entry-level nurse. To do this, about twelve thousand newly licensed nurses are interviewed on the frequency of their nursing care practice. They are also interviewed on the importance of these practices. A correlation is then drawn between the frequency of nursing care activities, their usefulness in maintaining client safety and their impact on a client's environment. Based on the results of the research, the board develops an exam structure that incorporates client needs and fundamental nursing processes.

Pass Rates

In 26 years, more than 5.7 million people have taken the NCLEX. The national first-time pass rate for nurses in 2018 was 88%. The NCSBN publishes quarterly and yearly pass rates on a national and school level. Regardless of this, a candidate's chances of passing aren't dependent on school or nationality, but on individual preparation and effort.

About seven in ten test-takers pass the exam. Pass rates vary widely between first-time takers and repeat takers, and also between US-educated nurses and international nursing school graduates.

How to Register for the NCLEX-RN

The process to register for the NCLEX-RN exam can be broken down into four steps:

Application – First, submit an application to the state board of nursing where you wish to obtain a license. For example, if you went to a nursing school in Michigan and wish to get your registered nursing license in Michigan, then you have to apply to the state board of nursing in Michigan. On the other hand, if you went to a nursing school in Oklahoma and wish to get your nursing license in New York, then you have to apply to the state board of nursing in New York. After getting your license in your preferred state, if you wish to work in a different state altogether, all you need to do is apply to that state board of nursing. You don't need to retake the licensing exam. Note that each state has individual requirements for eligibility. You must meet the requirements of your preferred state to be eligible for the exam.

Registration – After getting clearance from your preferred nursing board, you can register for the exam via Pearson VUE's website. Your nursing school should provide you with any required forms and assist you with the necessary information for registration.

Authorization – After registration, Pearson VUE will send you an Authorization to Test (ATT). The ATT has information like your test authorization number, candidate number and validity date. You should take your test within the validity date, which is an average of 90 days. Pearson VUE does not offer extension dates. If you don't take the exams before the validity date expires, you will need to start the registration process all over again.

Scheduling – You will have to schedule a testing appointment at Pearson VUE. This includes choosing your preferred date, location and time. This appointment can be made online or by phone. After that, you will receive an email confirming your appointment with directions to the exam center of your choice.

If, for some reason, you wish to change your exam appointment, you can do so. However, if you fail to cancel your appointment and miss the test, you will need to start the registration process again. To change an exam appointment, contact Pearson VUE either through their website or by phone. You must do this at least 24 hours before your appointment date and time. For example, if your exam is scheduled for noon on Friday, you must contact Pearson VUE no later than 12 p.m. Thursday.

Payment

You can pay to register for the test using a credit card, prepaid card or debit Mastercard. The registration fee is a flat fee of $200. There are no additional payments except when you request a change of state nursing board, after registering an initial one. There are no refunds for any of these fees. If you do not receive confirmation of your NCLEX registration two days after submitting your application, contact the NCLEX Candidate Service. Do not submit another application or pay another registration fee before calling.

NCLEX-RN Exam Fees

Fee	NCLEX Candidate Seeking Licensure
Registration fee	$200
Additional international scheduling fee with VAT where applicable	$150
Change the nursing regulatory body after the registration fee	$50
Change exam language (English/French) after registration fee	Not applicable

NCLEX Test Dates and Exam Centre

NCLEX-RN test dates are available all year round. First-time takers are offered test dates that fall within thirty days of their request, while repeat takers are offered test dates that fall within 45 days of their request. You should schedule a test date as soon as possible, to increase your chances of getting good test dates and locations. Many people take this test annually. Unnecessary delays can put you at risk of having to register again, particularly when your ATT expires.

There are NCLEX exam centers all over the United States and Canada. This variety of options means you can take your exam at a location that will most likely be convenient for you. However, if the center is outside the country where you seek to be licensed, you will be charged additional fees.

For candidates seeking licensure in the US and Australia, domestic testing centers are located within the US and its territories. For those seeking licensure in Canada, domestic testing centers are located in Canada and its territories and also in the US, excluding its territories.

International test centers are subject to change without notice. However, candidates will be informed of the change and encouraged to reschedule the exam at another center. If a candidate wishes to reschedule the exam to a domestic center, charges for the international scheduling will be refunded.

NCLEX-RN Retake Policies

According to the NCSBN, you can take an exam no more than eight times in one year. However, there is no limitation to the number of retakes for an applicant. That said, be aware some state nursing boards have strict retake policies:

Kansas – Candidates seeking licensure in Kansas have two years from their date of graduation to do so. After two years, they have to submit a petition for permission to retest.

Louisiana – Candidates seeking licensure in Louisiana have up to four years from their date of graduation to do so. In those four years, candidates can take the exam up to four times.

Michigan – Michigan allows applicants to retake the exam a maximum of six times, total, and not more than three times a year. If candidates don't pass the exam in the first three attempts, they have to take a board-approved education program. After the program, they are allowed to make the last three attempts.

South Carolina – Candidates who fail at their first attempt are given another attempt that should be taken no more than a year from the last test. If candidates don't pass after that, they must take a board-certified remedial course before retaking the exam. If candidates don't pass by the third year of their graduation, they are required to attend a nursing education program before taking the test again.

NCLEX-RN EXAM DAY

What You Need

Mental State – A positive mental attitude is the first requirement for any worthwhile venture. If you are retaking the test, it may not be easy to hope for the best, when you've been faced with previous failure, but it can be done. Visualization and affirmation of a favorable outcome may be useful. It can also help if you lean on the support of friends, family and mentors.

Dress Comfortably – Hats, scarves, gloves and coats aren't allowed into the exam room. However, provisions are made for religious and cultural attire. Your clothes should be comfortable and appropriate. This not only improves your mood but saves you from distractions and delays. Students must wear a mask and gloves during the exam as per NCSBN's guidelines.

Punctuality – Apart from being in a calm and peaceful state of mind, you should arrive at your test center at least thirty minutes before the exam time. You will need that time to have your identification processed. Here are some tips to help you show up on time:

1. After receiving your ATT, schedule your test as early as possible.
2. Choose testing centers that are close to your residential area.
3. Choose testing centers in familiar areas.
4. If your testing center is located in an unfamiliar area, do a test drive before the test day.
5. If your testing center is far away, consider staying in a hotel or at a friend's place.
6. It is very important to choose a test date and time that is convenient for you.
7. Go to bed early the day before. The night before your exam isn't an ideal time for all-night reading, coffee-binging or staying up late with friends.
8. Set an alarm if you are a deep sleeper.
9. You should factor in the weather and traffic before deciding the appropriate time to leave the house.
10. Finally, it is better to be too early than to be too late.

What to Do

Check-In – Electronic devices are not allowed in the test room. Cell phones, smartphones, tablets and other electronic devices are stored in sealable plastic bags and secured in a locker. Candidates who refuse to store their electronic devices are disqualified from taking the exam.

Identification – At the center, you are expected to show an authorized ID to confirm your identity. This ID's name should match the name used to register for the exam. It should also have a photograph and your signature. A second ID is needed if the first ID doesn't have a signature. In this case, the signature should match the name on the ATT and the secondary ID.

If you change your name after obtaining your ATT, you will need to bring documents that prove your change of name. Acceptable documents are a marriage license, a divorce record and court papers concerning your name change. Acceptable identification includes a driver's license, a passport, a permanent residence card with a recent photo or a military identification card. On arrival, test administrators take you through a formal check-in process for verification. The verification process includes:

First, you present your authorized form of personal identification to the administrator, who confirms its validity.

Next, a photograph of you is taken and a digital copy is made of your signature. Your palm is given a biometric scan.

Seating Arrangements – After verification, you are ushered into the exam room and assigned your designated seat and computer. The exam environment is roomy, calm, quiet and comfortable. The temperature is adapted to suit the time of the year. You shouldn't leave the seat except for breaks and when you are done with the exams.

The exam room not only accommodates NCLEX-RN exam-takers but a host of other exam-takers whose questions may include essay questions. Keyboard clicks, coughs and sneezes are usual sounds. If you find these sounds distracting, you can always ask for earplugs. Apart from earplugs, an erasable board and a marker are provided for making calculations.

NCLEX-RN Test Accommodations – Accommodations are provided for people with hearing, visual and other impairments. Some of these accommodations include extra test time, a separate room with a reader, a screen magnifier, a separate room with a sign language interpreter, a hearing aid and a separate room with a recorder.

NCLEX-RN Test Accommodation Requirements

Not everyone qualifies for test accommodations. For example, candidates with English as a second language are not eligible for accommodations. Candidates with anxiety disorders, sexual disorders, gambling addictions and substance abuse disorders are also not eligible for accommodations.

State boards follow standardized guidelines to screen candidates who apply for accommodations. For example, Louisiana uses the Diagnostic and Statistical Manual (DSM) and also the American Disabilities Act (ADA) guidelines. You should refer to your nursing board for information on guidelines for eligibility.

How to Apply for Accommodations

To apply for a testing accommodation, refer to your nursing board. After making the necessary inquiries, you should submit a written application requesting a test accommodation.

Although requirements vary from state to state, supporting documents to prove eligibility are always required. Examples of such documents include a formal recommendation from your school's dean or the director of your nursing program, attesting that similar accommodations were made for you in the past. You will also need to provide your medical records and a medical report by the medical professional who attends to your condition.

If you are approved for testing accommodations, contact Pearson VUE either by phone or by mail before registration. Candidates who have been granted an accommodation should contact the NCLEX-RN Accommodations Coordinator to schedule their tests.

NCLEX-RN Exam Rules and Regulations

Candidates are required to review the NCLEX rules before commencing the exam. On the exam day, candidates must read the candidate statement and agree to the terms and conditions.

Security

1. Personal effects are placed in individual storage lockers.
2. Candidates are recorded by audio and visual cameras.
3. The exam administrators are not liable for any missing or stolen items.
4. The following items are banned during the entire duration of the exam, including during the verification process and lunch-breaks: any form of study materials, electronics like smartphones, tablets, MP3 players, Bluetooth earpieces, fitness bands, cameras and the like. Weapons are also prohibited.
5. Sealable plastic bags are provided for storing electronic devices. After the exam, candidates are expected to return the bags.
6. The following items aren't allowed in the testing room but can be accessed during breaks: coats, hats, gloves, scarves, food or drink, lip balm, cosmetics, medical aids/devices, wallets, bags, purses and non-smart watches.

Conduct and Confidentiality – Candidates are not permitted to bring a second party to the exam center.

1. Candidates are not permitted to ask for help in answering questions, whether in person or by mail, text or phone calls. This restriction includes during the exam, during lunch breaks and after the exam.
2. Candidates are not permitted to discuss questions with anyone, including instructors and study group members. Nor are they allowed to post and discuss questions on the internet.
3. Candidates are not permitted to remove items used for the exam, including boards, board markers and earplugs.
4. Candidates are not allowed to copy the exam questions for any reason.

Test Administration

1. Candidates cannot take the exam on behalf of anybody. No one can take the exam on your behalf.
2. Candidates are not permitted to use the testing center computers for any reason apart from what they are intended for.
3. Candidates are not permitted to disrupt the examination or act as a distraction to others.
4. Boards and erasable markers are provided for the examination.
5. Candidates are not allowed to use the board for any reason apart from what it was intended for.
6. Writing on any other material apart from the board is prohibited.
7. Candidates are expected to return the board and marker after the exam is over.

8. Candidates are allowed to notify the test administrator of any hardware or software challenges during the exam. They can do so by raising a hand.
9. Earplugs are provided on request. Personal earplugs are prohibited.

Break Sessions

1. The first scheduled break is given after two hours of the exam.
2. Unscheduled breaks are allowed for emergencies. Candidates are permitted to signal a request for an unscheduled break by raising their hands. The exam timer doesn't stop during scheduled or unscheduled breaks.
3. Candidates are not permitted to engage the test administrator in any informal or formal conversation before, during and after the examination. Any questions about the exam should be directed to the NCSBN.

Dismissal or Cancelation of Results

1. Candidates who violate the test center rules and regulations may be dismissed from the exam. There are no refunds for the examination fee.
2. Other sanctions may include cancelation of the exam and further disciplinary actions from your state nursing board. These sanctions may include denial of a license, denial of future registration and disqualification from future licensure.
3. Disruptive and unacceptable behaviors include, but are not limited to:

   Using or attempting to access prohibited aids. Examples of prohibited aids include electronic gadgets, calculators, conversion tables, dictionaries, study materials and so on.
   - Disobeying the instructions of the test administrator.
   - Disruption of any kind.

- Impersonation on behalf of someone else, or having someone impersonate you.
- Giving or receiving assistance during the exam.
- Attempting to use the computer for another function apart from the exam.

Length of the Exam

The NCLEX-RN exam is a computerized adaptive test. This test format excludes the need for oral and theory questions. Tests used to range from 75 to 265 questions, but the pandemic has caused some changes. Now the questions will range from 60 to a maximum of 130 questions. Test takers must answer at least 60 questions correctly to pass the exam. The pretest questions have been removed in 2020 and will not show up on the exam as per NCSBN's new guidelines. You are given a maximum of four hours to complete the exam. These four hours include a short tutorial on the exams, one or two scheduled breaks and other unscheduled breaks. The test used to be six hours long but has been reduced to four hours due to the pandemic, at the time of writing this book. These rules may change in the future.

Based on your performance, the testing can be longer or shorter. This means that the test stops when the algorithm decides if you have met or failed the passing standard. The test also stops when all the questions are answered or when the six-hour limit is up. To increase your chances of success, you should maintain a steady pace during the test, which is roughly about two minutes per question. At the end of the exam, you are required to answer a brief survey questionnaire that quizzes you on your exam experience, from the time you check in to the point you stop your exam. You are also required to signal your completion of the exam by raising your hand. At this point, the test administrator will retrieve all the materials given to you for the examination.

Getting Test Results

Each NCLEX-RN exam is scored twice for quality control, once by the computer algorithm in the test center, and once by the algorithm at Pearson VUE. However, results aren't released at the exam center. Results are sent to your nursing board and to your email approximately six weeks after the examination.

However, some states allow their candidates to access their results after 48 working days. This access is granted through the quick results service. This service is not available for candidates seeking licensure in Canada and Australia. Candidates are not permitted to contact Pearson VUE NCLEX Candidate Service, the test administrators or the NCSBN for exam results. If you do not get your test results in more than six weeks, contact your nursing board.

Test Cancelation

The NCSBN has high standards that give candidates opportunities to demonstrate their strengths while also preventing any bias. Because of this, the NCSBN has the authority to cancel or withhold a result when a test violates its principles. Examples of such scenarios include:

1. There is a testing irregularity.
2. There is a falsification and/or impersonation.
3. A test-taker is involved in misconduct, inappropriate and/or irregular behavior.
4. A test-taker violates the confidentiality agreement.

5. The test is judged to be invalid for any other reason, even when there is no evidence of a candidate's involvement in irregularities.
6. Invalid results may take the form of an unusual score or unusual answer patterns.

Cancelation Appeal

If your result is canceled or withheld without substantial evidence of your personal involvement in irregularities, you can appeal the NCSBN decision, and you will be offered a free retest.

Candidate Performance Report

Candidates who fail the exam are sent a two-page candidate performance report. This NCLEX CPR is individualized and sent to candidates who fail to answer at least 60 questions. The number of questions answered indicates how close a candidate was to the passing standard. Candidates whose score was close to the passing standard will answer about 130 questions. Candidates whose score was further away from the passing standard will answer fewer questions. The NCLEX-RN exam is not graded in sections. Pass or fail status is determined by performance across all sections.

The report tells you how many questions were answered and how many were left for evaluation. The front page of the CPR contains a brief summary of how the CAT works. It also summarizes how many questions were answered and provides guidelines on how to use the information provided on the second page. On the second page, there is a breakdown of a candidate's performance on the NCLEX test content areas. These content areas are grouped into Below the Passing Standard, Near the Passing Standard and Above the Passing Standard.

Each of these content areas is described with percentages and a list of topics related to the area. These descriptions are used as references to assess areas of weaknesses. They are also used as guides for future retakes.

A good way to use the performance report is to prioritize the areas covered in Below the Passing Standard, then move on to those listed in Near the Passing Standard and Above the Passing Standard. The NCLEX CPR is not a prediction of a candidate's future outcome. It only indicates a candidate's strengths and weaknesses.

NCLEX-RN Exam Structure

The NCLEX-RN is a computerized-adaptive testing (CAT) exam. CAT is an advanced software algorithm that uses information technology and modern cognitive measurements to make exams efficient and individualized.

How CAT Works

When you answer a question, the computer algorithm assesses your ability and efficiency by analyzing the data from previous answers and the difficulty of previous questions. From this analysis, the algorithm then selects the next question that has a 50% probability of being answered correctly. As more questions are answered, the algorithm assesses your ability and selects questions that are increasingly difficult or easy, depending on your previous performance. This process continues until the algorithm has assessed your level of competence.

There are no provisions to skip a question. One question appears at a time on the screen. You are allowed to take as long as you want on each question. However, the question must be answered before the next question is displayed. Because of this, you can be tempted to take wild guesses at difficult questions. Wild guesses are not advisable. You should select the best possible answer. There is also a temptation to spend a longer time on difficult questions. This is also not advisable. Although you are expected to answer as many questions correctly as possible, you should answer the test questions at a steady and timed pace.

Benefits of a CAT-Based NCLEX-RN Exam

Individualization – CAT-based exams are tailored to match your ability. This feature eliminates bias and promotes fairness. For example, high-performing candidates are challenged with increasingly complex questions. Conversely, lower-performing candidates aren't overloaded with difficult questions which may cause them to give up quickly.

Precision – CAT-based exams use reliable methods to precisely measure your ability in relation to nursing skills and proficiency.

Security – Since questions are chosen from a pool of questions, the chances of CAT exam malpractice and other security concerns are reduced.

How the Questions Will Appear

Most of the questions in the NCLEX-RN are multiple-choice. However, there are other formats too. These formats include multiple responses, fill in the blanks, ordered response, hotspot, figures, charts, graphics, audio and video.

Multiple-Choice Questions

This is the most common format used in the NCLEX-RN exam. In this format, candidates are given text-based questions about a clinical scenario. The candidate can only select one of four answer options. Multiple-choice questions are not only used for text-based questions but also for charts, audio and graphics.

Chart Question Format

This is also called an exhibit question format. The question is a chart which is supported by four options. The candidate can only select one correct option.

Graphic Question Format

In this format, the question is in text form. The supporting options are in the form of pictures. The candidate is expected to select the correct picture.

Audio Question Format

In this format, the candidate is given a question in audio form. The question is followed by four text-based answer options. The candidate is expected to click on the audio icon, listen to the audio with headphones and choose the correct option. The candidate can listen to the audio as many times as necessary.

Video Question Format

In this format, the candidate is given a question in video form. This question is followed by four text-based answer options. The candidate is expected to view the video clip and select the correct option.

Select All That Apply Question Format

In this format, the candidate is required to select all the text-based options that answer questions. There are usually more than four options in this type of question. Partial credit is not given in this question format, i.e., the candidate must select all the correct options in order for the question to be counted as correct.

Fill-in-the-Blank Question Format

This format is typically used for drug calculations, calculating intravenous flow rate and fluid output and input. In this format, the student solves the problem and fills in the correct answer.

Ordered Response Question Format

In this format, the candidate is given a question in a text-based form. This question is preceded by text-based options that should be arranged in order.

Hotspot Text-Based Question Format

In this format, the candidate is given a picture. This picture is followed by a text-based question. The candidate is expected to click on a specific area.

NCLEX-RN Passing Standard

The NCSBN's Board of Directors reevaluates its passing standard every three years. Because the nursing practice is subject to change, it is important to use passing standards that are accurate and reflect the current nursing skills required to practice as an entry-level registered nurse. In evaluating a passing standard, the board organizes a comprehensive review on factors like:

1. The results of a standardized exam are analyzed and assessed by a panel of qualified judges. Statistical results that comprise procedures and criterion-referenced standard-setting methods are used.

2. An assessment of the historical record of the passing standard and annual summaries of candidates' performance on the NCLEX CAT.

3. Results from yearly surveys done by employers and educators. The aim of these surveys is to get practical opinions on the current and expected competence of an entry-level registered nurse.

4. An analysis of the readiness of high-school graduates who are interested in becoming nurses.

In December 2018, the NCSBN Board of Directors decided to maintain the current NCLEX-RN passing standard at 0.00 logits. This decision is valid until March 31, 2022.

Definition of Terms

Candidate Ability – The level of nursing knowledge, skills and ability of a candidate.

Ability Estimate – The level of skills, knowledge and ability the computer algorithm estimates a candidate has.

Passing Standard – The minimum ability level required of an entry-level nurse.

Logit – A unit of measurement used to report relative differences between a candidate's ability and question difficulty.

Pass/Fail Rules

The computer algorithm uses a system to decide if a candidate has passed or failed the NCLEX-RN exam. Candidates are assessed using one of these three rules;

95% Confidence Interval Rule – In this rule, the computer stops giving the candidate test questions when it is 95% sure that the candidate's ability is above the passing standard or below the passing standard.

Maximum Length Exam – This rule is used for a candidate whose ability is close to the passing standard. In this rule, the computer continues to give test questions until it reaches the maximum number of test questions. In this rule, the computer algorithm assesses your status by your final ability estimate, meaning that a passing score is given if your final ability estimate is above the passing standard and vice versa.

Run Out of Time Rule – This rule is used for candidates who run out of time before the computer algorithm assesses their performance. In this rule, a candidate fails if he/she was unable to answer the minimum number of questions. However, if the candidate answers the minimum number of questions, the computer reviews the last 60 questions. If the candidate's ability estimate was above the passing standard, a passing score is awarded. If the candidate's ability dropped below the passing standard, the candidate has failed the exam.

Tips on How to Pass the NCLEX-RN Exam

Passing the NCLEX-RN exam is a combination of preparation, organization and mental attitude.

Preparation

Adequate preparation has a lot to do with the type of materials you prepare with, the amount of time you spend preparing and the capacity of your recall.

How to Choose the Right Study Materials

Here are a few things to consider before choosing the right study material for your exams:

1. **Relevance** – Your study material should be relevant to the exam. This tip may be obvious, but there are lots of study materials that aren't relevant to the NCLEX-RN exam. To increase your chances of selecting relevant study material, you can buy resources that are recommended by your tutors, colleagues and peers who have passed the exams.

2. **Revised** – How current is your study material? The NCSBN reviews the NCLEX-RN exam every three years; therefore, your study material should be current, updated and revised to reflect the NCSBN standards. To increase your chances of selecting relevant study materials, you should also get recommendations from tutors, colleagues and successful candidates.

3. **Cost** – Beware of outrageously expensive materials that can put a dent in your pocket. There are decent materials that are reasonably priced and affordable; you just need to know where to obtain them.

4. **Highlights** – Your study material should give highlights on the distribution of test questions and priority areas to focus on. The right study material should help you narrow your studies to key areas.

5. **Comprehensive Rationales** – Your study material should give a comprehensive rationale for test questions and their answers. This fine-tunes your critical thinking and helps you identify subtle words and distinctions you didn't notice before.

6. **Organized** – Your study material should be organized methodically. Study materials that break down broad topics into outlines and sections improve a candidate's recall. Haphazard study materials can slow your preparation process.

How Much Time Should You Spend Studying?

It depends on you. There is no one-size-fits-all plan of study. But there are a few basic factors that can help you determine how long you should study.

1. **Start Early** – Early preparation increases your chances of success because you have time for study, experimentation and mistakes. Yes, you can make mistakes in your studying, especially if you are taking the exam for the first time. You can start out with the wrong resource material, or your study plan can be inefficient.

Whatever the error, early preparation gives you room to revise and adjust your study plan.

2. **Have a Study Goal** – Although the aim of your study session is to pass your NCLEX-RN exam, you will need a study goal to help you achieve this. Remember, your goal must be SMART: specific, measurable, achievable, relevant and time-bound.

For example, let's say you have a study goal to review the 400 questions in this book in a month. This goal has met three requirements of the SMART goal. It is specific, measurable and time-bound. You will have to determine how many questions you can answer in a day, how much time will be allotted to each study session and whether the amount of time you have available makes this a feasible goal.

3. **Create a Study Schedule** – A study schedule can be helpful to ensure you meet your study goals. For example, let's say you plan to cover the 400 questions in this study guide within a month. Your next step will be to create a detailed study schedule that shows how much time is allocated to each study session. A plan helps you track your progress and keeps you disciplined and focused.

4. **Choose the Suitable Study Method** – You should be familiar with your study methods and stick to them. Once you find something that works for you, don't change it. For example, students always ask if they should study alone or in a group. Group studying has its advantages and disadvantages, and so does studying solo. The truth is that neither study method is better than the other. Some candidates study efficiently on their own, while some do better in groups. A good tip is to use both forms of study, devoting more time to your dominant study method. That way, you can harness the benefits of both study methods.

5. **Extracurricular Activities** – You should factor rest, sleep, breaks and physical activity into your study schedule.

How to Improve Your Recall

Recall is an important aspect of studying. After all, what's the point of studying if you can't recall significant information when you need to? Here are a few tips to improve your recall:

1. **Read Actively** – Here are a few tips to help you read actively:

A. Read with a Focus – By giving you specific areas to focus on, study materials increase your engagement and concentration.

B. Take Notes As You Read – As you read, you can make notes, create mnemonics, questions or a to-do post-reading list. You can also highlight sections that you know you will need to review in more detail.

C. Take Breaks – Active reading requires focus and effort, and if done correctly, it can't be done over a long stretch of time. For example, it is advised that study sessions be kept to a range of two to three hours. Anything longer, and you may struggle to concentrate.

2. **Study in a Group** – Group study can improve recall because group study is an effective form of studying large quantities of test questions.

3. **Use Mnemonics** – Mnemonics are great tools for improving your recall. However, they should be used only after understanding the concepts of the topic you read. Mnemonics include but are not limited to acronyms, rhymes, imagery, chunking and use of loci.

4. **Understand First Principles** – Nursing is a science that is based on facts, logic and reasoning. Understanding topics from a first-principle basis improves

your ability to store and retrieve information. When studying, always try to link the information together, building on your knowledge methodically.

5. **Sleep** – Sleep consolidates short-term memory. As you study, do not skip sleep. An adult requires an average of seven to nine hours of sleep a night. Therefore, when you create your study plan, factor in your need to get adequate sleep.

How to be Organized

To increase your chances of success, you should organize your activities before and during the exam.

1. **Early Registration** – We discussed the importance of early registration in chapter 2. Early registration increases your chances of success because it switches you into study mode. Early registration also gives you room to cope with unforeseen circumstances.

2. **Punctuality** – Always aim to show up at least 30 minutes early to the exam center. This gives you time to verify your identity, acquaint yourselves with the rules of the center and adjust to the environment.

3. **Dressing** – Dress comfortably and professionally. Remember that coats are not allowed into the exam hall. If you get cold easily, don't wear clothes made with thin fabric.

Tips on Answering Select-All-that-Apply Questions

Each option can either be true or false, but never both. Treating each option as true or false increases your chances of success.

Tips on Answering Fill-in-the-Blank Questions

A. Be sure to carefully read and follow the instructions shown on the screen.

B. Use the on-screen calculator provided.

C. Type in the figure you got from your calculation, and leave out any signs or symbols.

D. Round up your answers only at the end of the calculation.

Tips on Answering Ordered-Response Questions

These questions are usually about nursing procedures. Imagine yourself as a nurse in the clinical scenario.

Tips on Answering Hotspot Questions

This question format is used for questions on human anatomy, physiology and pathophysiology. Try to locate anatomic landmarks to increase your chances of answering the question correctly.

Having the Right Mental Attitude

A positive mental attitude is important for taking the NCLEX-RN exam, particularly for candidates retaking the exam. If you don't have a positive mental attitude, it is unlikely you will prepare properly for the exam, much less pass the test. Here are a few tips to improve your mental attitude:

1. **Study Group Peers** – You can get support from your study group peers who share the same goal with you.

2. **Tutors and Mentors** – You can also get support and encouragement from your tutors and mentors.

3. **Successful Candidates** – Successful candidates give you practical information and insight to help you succeed.

4. **Visualization and Affirmation** – These tools are great to boost your confidence and improve your attitude towards the exam.

5. **Sleep** – Adequate rest can improve your mood, attitude and cognitive functions.

Chapter 2: The Integrated Processes of the NCLEX-RN

There are five integrated processes assessed during the NCLEX-RN exam. These processes are the building blocks of nursing practice. They are the nursing process, caring, communication/documentation, teaching/ learning and culture/spirituality.

The Nursing Process

According to the NCSBN, nursing processes are defined as "the scientific, clinical reasoning approach to client care that includes assessment, analysis, planning, implementation and evaluation."

The nursing process used by RNs is substantially different from the nursing process of a practical nurse (LPN). The nursing process used by an LPN uses the principles of data collection, planning, implementation and evaluation. On the other hand, an RN employs all these methods but goes further to use these principles as a building block to critical thinking, problem-solving and providing professional nursing care to clients. The nursing process of an RN is a holistic, ongoing and dynamic approach to client care. It includes assessment, diagnosis, planning, implementation and evaluation.

Assessment – The assessment phase is the first phase of the nursing process. This phase begins during the initial contact with the client. This assessment is not static, but dynamic, continuing throughout the client's care. An initial assessment is done at the first presentation, then reassessments/ongoing assessments are done throughout the client's care. Assessment requires good critical thinking skills, observation and collection of both objective and subjective data.

Subjective data is intangible values of mood, emotions, culture, spirituality, society and psychology. Objective data is tangible physiological data such as respiration, blood pressure, height, weight, urine output and others. Data can be collected from the client, caregivers, family and friends. Data can also be current or retrospective. Current data is useful for assessing a client's current clinical status. Retrospective data includes previous clinical history from medical records and is useful for gaining insight on past medical conditions and their management.

Data can also be primary or secondary. Primary data is obtained directly from clients, while secondary data is obtained from third parties like caregivers, relatives and friends. Quantitative data is numerical. Examples include a client's vital signs, fluid volume and laboratory values. Qualitative data is non-numerical. Examples include radiology films, their corresponding reports and microbiology culture reports.

Diagnosis – This phase involves the use of clinical and critical reasoning skills to assess a client's risk factors, challenges and possible solutions. The North American Nursing Diagnosis Association (NANDA) compiled an up-to-date list of nursing diagnoses. According to NANDA, a nursing diagnosis is "a clinical judgment about responses to actual or potential health problems in a patient, family or community."

To diagnose effectively, an RN has to prioritize client care according to needs and patient-centered outcomes. To do so, a nurse uses Maslow's Hierarchy of Needs. This hierarchy is based on the provision of basic and fundamental human needs. For example, basic physiological needs for water and food must be met before higher needs are addressed.

Maslow's Hierarchy of Needs

Basic Physiological Needs – Water, food, airway, breathing, circulation, excretion, sleep, sex, exercise and shelter.

Safety and Security – Prevention of injuries, hand hygiene, infection control, suicide precautions, safety precautions and primary prevention methods.

Love and Belonging – Provision of supportive relationships, reflective listening, therapeutic communication and sexual intimacy.

Self Esteem – Acceptance, personal achievement, self-acceptance and empowerment.

Self-Actualization – Spiritual growth, self-mastery, assertiveness and empowering environment.

There are different kinds of nursing diagnoses. Examples include actual diagnoses, wellness diagnoses, risk diagnoses, possible nursing diagnoses and syndrome nursing diagnoses. The components of a good nursing diagnosis include a problem, a qualifier, the cause of the need and the characteristics of the health care need.

Planning – In this phase, nursing care plans are created, giving direction for individual care provided to patients. A nursing plan should be unique to the client's needs and subject to evaluation and adjustments. A nursing plan should also be updated to suit the client's response to treatment.

Planning can be an initial plan, an ongoing plan or a discharge plan. Initial planning is the first plan created during an initial assessment of the client. An ongoing plan is done throughout the course of the client's care. This planning is dynamic and should reflect the current status of the client. A discharge plan is created when the client is discharged from the health facility. This plan is not a termination of medical care, but a continuum.

The planning phase involves goal-setting. The nurse creates goals that are tailored to provide professional and adequate patient care. These goals are directed by set guidelines and done in collaboration with the clients, their caregivers and other members of the health team. A goal should be SMART: specific, measurable, attainable, realistic and timely.

Implementation – In this step, nursing interventions are carried out in line with the nurse's assessment of data, diagnosis, priority of care and nursing care plan. To do this, the registered nurse must use skills like critical thinking, clinical judgment, problem-solving, priority setting and technical skills.

Nursing interventions can be dependent or independent interventions. A dependent intervention is done with a doctor's order, such as the administration of medications. Independent nursing interventions are done without a doctor's order. For example, turning and positioning of a client, assisting with feeding, dressing and bathing.

Evaluation – In this phase, current data is collated and compared to the client's initial data at presentation. After comparing the two, nursing care plans and interventions are adjusted to suit the expected goal. The evaluation phase of the nursing process must be performed by a registered nurse. The registered nurse is responsible for evaluating data collated by nursing assistants and LPNs. An RN is also responsible for making the necessary adjustments needed to achieve the desired therapeutic outcome. This is because the evaluation phase requires clinical reasoning and judgment skills that are beyond the scope of nursing assistants and LPNs.

For example, an RN monitors the respiration of a client with a tracheostomy by assessing the client's respiratory rate, heart rate, temperature and movement of the anterior chest wall. The RN also uses a stethoscope to listen to breath sounds.

A nursing care plan for such a client would include maintaining a patent airway, preventing infection, providing tracheostomy care and providing other means of communication. If the client goes into respiratory distress, the RN assesses the possible cause of the distress and institutes an intervention, such as encouraging the client to cough to expectorate secretions and suctioning the secretions. The RN does a reassessment of the client's respiration. If the client is still in distress, the RN does another reassessment to identify the possible cause of the distress and then initiates a new nursing intervention, such as providing warm, humidified supplementary oxygen.

Caring

Caring is the second component of the integrated process of the NCLEX-RN. According to the NCSBN, caring is "the interaction between the nurse and client, in an atmosphere of mutual respect and trust." This atmosphere nurtures the nurse-client relationship and makes it easy for the nurse to encourage, support and show compassion. Caring is not only shown to individuals but to groups, families and communities.

Concepts of Caring

Compassion – A person's emotional capacity to share in someone's distress, with a desire to alleviate it.

Empathy – The ability to stand in a speaker's shoes, see things from the speaker's perspective and communicate to the speaker that his/her emotions have been understood.

Sympathy – The ability to perceive another person's distress. Action to alleviate the distress may or may not be taken.

Altruism – In the clinical setting, altruism is a voluntary and selfless action taken by a health worker to improve the welfare of a client. These actions are usually not remunerated.

Sometimes, there may be no clear-cut line dividing all the concepts of care. An RN can be sympathetic and compassionate at the same time. In other cases, compassion can motivate an RN to be altruistic and vice versa.

The Theory of Human Care

Nursing theorist Jean Watson developed her Theory of Human Caring from 1975-1979. She drew inspiration from research, personal experiences and knowledge as a nursing educator to create a nursing theory that is known as the 10 Carative Factors:

1. Forming humanistic-altruistic value systems

2. Instilling faith and hope

3. Cultivating sensitivity to self and others

4. Developing a helping-trust relationship

5. Promoting an expression of feelings

6. Using problem-solving for decision-making

7. Promoting teaching-learning

8. Promoting a supportive environment

9. Assisting with the gratification of human needs

10. Allowing for existential-phenomenological forces.

Communication

Communication in nursing involves all the verbal and nonverbal interactions between a nurse and a client, members of the client's family and other members of the health team.

Communication can be verbal, as seen in a conversation between a nurse and the client. It can be nonverbal, as seen in demeanor, body language and mood. It can be written or pictorial. Whatever form of communication is used, it is important that the purpose of communication is met.

Components of Communication

Communication is a dynamic and ongoing process that involves a sender, information, receiver and response/feedback.

The Importance of Communication

As social beings, we do not only need food, water and shelter to survive. We also need to interact and communicate with one another. Here are a few reasons why we need to communicate.

To Share Information – Our brains are constantly processing the sensory information they receive. This information influences our actions, whether consciously or subconsciously. In a health-care setting, information is a crucial aspect of management and client care.

For Self-Expression – Communication helps us express our thoughts, feelings and emotions to others. Self-expression is gratifying and is an effective tool for easing tension and inner conflict.

For Support and Belonging – As social beings, humans are driven by a need to be accepted. Communication is necessary for support, acceptance and belonging. As we express our feelings and emotions to others, it becomes easy for others to understand, trust and accept us. Likewise, when we give people the opportunity to express themselves to us, it becomes easier for them to trust us.

Therapeutic Communication

In the nursing practice, therapeutic communication is a meaningful nurse-client interaction that helps improve the medical outcome of the client. Therapeutic communication is an active process that requires effort and attention from both the speaker and the listener. There are therapeutic communication techniques that are used to facilitate the communication process. On the other hand, there are roadblocks to therapeutic communication.

Therapeutic Communication Techniques

Silence – In this technique, the listener uses deliberate silence to give the speaker opportunity to express himself. The results of this technique are diverse. Deliberate silence eases tension, prevents conflicts, brings clarification and encourages self-expression.

Accepting – Accepting is not the same as giving compliments or flattery. When using this technique, the listener shows that he/she understands the speaker's emotions and affirms this to the speaker. The nurse may not support or agree with the client, but he/she acknowledges understanding.

Offering Self – This technique is used for nonverbal communication. An RN can offer time and attention to clients as a show of support. This can be as simple as keeping quiet to listen or staying behind after a shift to sit with a patient.

Giving recognition – Giving recognition is not the same as giving a compliment. In this technique, the listener acknowledges and draws attention to the actions of the speaker. This technique is useful for showing support and encouragement without using flattery or making judgments and evaluations.

Giving Broad Openings – This technique involves the use of open-ended questions. It allows the client to lead the conversation and direct the flow and mood of the conversation. An open question like "how are you today?" sets the pace for the client.

Making Observations – Using this technique, the nurse notices the client's demeanor, body language and facial expressions. This technique not only allows room for self-expression but is useful to help the nurse notice new symptoms.

Placing the Event in Time or Sequence – Using this technique, the nurse asks questions about the timing and occurrence of events. The aim is to get clarification and encourage the client to recall more information.

Focusing – Using this technique, the nurse focuses on important aspects of the client's conversation and encourages him/her to expound on certain things.

Reflecting – Reflection is important when a client is seeking an evaluation or a solution to a problem. The nurse can direct the problem back to the client by asking questions like, "What do you think you should do?" This makes the client responsible for his/her actions. It also improves self-awareness and reliance.

Paraphrasing – Using this technique, a nurse interprets the emotional content of a client's words and paraphrases the meaning back to show that what the person said has been understood. This technique encourages clarification and self-expression.

Encouraging Comparison – When using this technique, the nurse encourages the client to recall similar experiences. The aim of this technique is to encourage the client to think of solutions to challenges.

Active Listening – This technique utilizes prompts to engage and encourage the speaker to continue talking. It shows that the nurse is paying attention to the client. Examples of prompts include "Go on" and "I see."

Seeking Clarification – This technique is used by the nurse to clarify any confusion or ambiguity. It tells the client that the nurse is paying attention. A statement like "I don't understand what you said" is a good example of how to seek clarification.

Encouraging Description of Perception – The nurse uses this technique for clients experiencing sensory hallucinations. This technique is non-judgmental, non-evaluative and gives the client freedom for self-expression.

Voicing Doubt – This technique is used only after trust has been established. By expressing doubt, the nurse encourages the client to take responsibility.

Confronting – This technique must be used only after trust is established. If used incorrectly, this technique can become a roadblock to effective communication. But when used correctly, it can help clients to take responsibility.

Restating – This technique is used to show that the listener understands. The nurse repeats the exact words of the client to show that he/she was heard.

Encouraging Goal-Setting – The nurse uses this technique to encourage clients to be more involved and take responsibility. This technique requires tact because the nurse can unknowingly slip into evaluation and judgment.

Encouraging Formulation of Plan of Action – This technique should be used only after trust is established. The nurse encourages the client to think of possible solutions to challenges.

Limit Setting – This technique should be used after trust is established or when the client shows inappropriate behavior. The nurse discourages inappropriate behavior from the client and encourages appropriate conduct. For example, the nurse can say, "Please stop what you are doing. If you don't, I will leave."

Suggest Collaboration – Using this technique, the nurse offers help to the client. Note that offering unsolicited help can be a roadblock to therapeutic communication.

Non-Therapeutic Communication Techniques

Non-therapeutic communication techniques are roadblocks to effective communication. These techniques involve the use of words or phrases that make a patient feel defensive, threatened and uncomfortable.

Overloading – When using this technique, the speaker gives too much information. The speaker talks too fast or changes the subject matter too frequently. For example, a nurse who is overloading might ask a client, "Have you produced the sputum sample? Did you eat breakfast on time? Are you ready for the x-ray?"

False Reassurance – When using this technique, the nurse uses cliché statements to reassure the client. This technique makes the client feel like his/her concerns are invalid and trifle. An example of a cliché statement is, "You will be fine."

Focusing on Self – When using this technique, the nurse is focused on his/her needs and not the needs of the client.

Giving Advice – This technique should only be used after trust has been achieved. The nurse attempts to help the client by offering advice. The use of this technique implies that the nurse is taking responsibility for the client's actions.

Underloading – When using this technique, the nurse attempts to block communication by remaining mute, ignoring the client's cues for conversation and not responding to feedback.

Invalidation – When using this technique, the nurse ignores the mood of the client. For example, a client who wants to start a conversation may be shunned by a nurse who says he/she is too busy to talk.

Value Judgments – When using this technique, the nurse attempts to give his/her opinion and make a distinction between right and wrong.

Probing – When using this technique, the nurse asks leading questions in an attempt to know more so as to make a moral evaluation. This technique can cause the client to become defensive, uncomfortable and resentful.

Internal Validation – This technique can also be called jumping to conclusions. The listener is quick to make assumptions about the speaker's behavior without giving the speaker time to express emotions.

Stereotyping – When using this technique, the nurse uses blanket statements and cliché responses. This technique disregards the uniqueness of an individual.

Defensiveness – When using this technique, the nurse attempts to defend his/her actions or his/her colleagues' mistakes. This technique shifts the focus away from the client and is not therapeutic.

Changing the Subject – When using this technique, the nurse attempts to steer the conversation away from uncomfortable areas. This technique is not therapeutic because it shifts the focus away from the client.

Documentation

Documentation is an example of written communication. Examples of documents used in health facilities include medical records, health policies, procedures, care plans and investigation reports. Apart from transmitting messages, documents are used to process health insurance reimbursement. Documents are also used as proof of legal issues. Documentation is a mandatory requirement from any state's regulatory bodies.

Types of Medical Records

There are various methods used to document medical information. Each of these methods has its advantages and disadvantages. They include case management and critical pathways, focused charting, charting by exception, source-oriented medical records, the PIE method and problem-oriented medical records.

Case Management and Critical Pathways

This record system is relatively new. In this method, pre-planned care templates are created because it is assumed that most patients with specific medical and nursing diagnoses have a similar approach to care. These pre-planned templates are created via a collaborative effort by a multidisciplinary team. When a variance occurs, it is recorded and used in evaluation and improvement studies. Variance can be patient-related, provider-related or system-related.

Focused Charting

This form of documentation is not so popular. This method focuses on patient-related issues like diagnoses, challenges, strengths and conditions. Documentation is done in a three-columned form that contains a date and time of entry, a patient-related issue and a progress note. This method is easy to use.

However, it doesn't allow other health-care workers to include documentation, so information is scattered.

Charting by Exception

In this method, only abnormal and significant findings are documented. This method is rarely used because it is not an efficient method of capturing all important aspects of a client's data. For example, it is easy for health workers to assume that all abnormal data has been captured, when, in reality, health workers may have forgotten to record the data.

Source-Oriented Medical Record

This is one of the oldest methods of documentation. In this method, the client's data is kept in a metal flip chart. The client's records are divided into sections like laboratory, nursing, medical records, physical therapy and so on. This method is familiar and easy to use and follow. However, it is not multidisciplinary, and the client's information is scattered.

PIE (Problem, Intervention and Evaluation) Progress Notes

This method is compatible with other forms of medical documentation. In this method, the client's data is organized into problems, interventions done by a health worker and the results of the interventions. This method is familiar and easy to use.

Problem-Oriented Medical Record

This documentation method is multidisciplinary and organized. In this method, the client's records are arranged according to the client's problems. This is then attached to a section of the client's medical record. All members of the managing team compile and update a list of the client's problems and document the care that was given. This method encourages collaboration with other members of the managing team. However, it is unfamiliar and therefore difficult to utilize.

Teaching and Learning

An RN is also an educator. RNs are not only responsible for providing nursing care to clients, but they are also responsible for teaching clients, communities, nursing assistants and LPNs. RNs also conduct research and publish their findings in scholarly journals.

Clients – An RN educates a client on his/her medical condition, treatment options and nursing care plans. The aim is to keep the client involved in his/her care. An RN also educates the client on primary prevention methods and nursing interventions to make daily activities easier to keep up with.

Communities – An RN educates communities on ways to prevent disease. Some of these prevention methods include handwashing, vaccination, breastfeeding, environmental sanitation, food and water hygiene.

Nursing Assistants and Vocational Nurses – An RN is responsible for teaching nursing assistants and LPNs. Teaching concepts include data collection, documentation and evaluation.

Importance of Patient Education

Knowledge – A well-informed patient is empowered with sufficient information to make the right choices for his/her health. Also, a well-informed patient is more likely to cooperate with the health team.

Safety – A client who is informed of the primary prevention methods of his/her condition is likely to make the right choices to stay safe. Apart from that, the client can become an advocate for primary health prevention and educate family, friends and community.

Improved Patient Outcome – Clients who cooperate with the health team have better outcomes. They are quick to make decisions on medical treatments, procedures and treatment care plans. This can greatly improve the outcome, reduce complications and shorten hospital admissions.

Team Work – A client is also a part of the health team. Patient education is a core aspect of patient-centered care.

Learning Methods

Before an RN begins to educate a client, he/she must know the client's preferred and most effective learning method. A lot of patients do not have in-depth knowledge of their medical conditions.

To prevent misinterpretation and confusion, the RN should familiarize him/herself with the client's learning methods and adjust teaching strategies accordingly. A good way to do so is to ask the client his/her preferred learning method. This may include any of the following:

Visual Method – Includes the use of educational videos, models, pictures, flow charts, diagrams and demonstrations.

Verbal Method – The use of spoken and written communication, such as in presentations, and the use of audiotapes.

Auditory Method – The use of recorded tapes, music and audio files.

Tactile Method – Involves hands-on experience, as seen in role-playing and demonstrations.

Obstacles to Effective Learning

Language – It is difficult to teach clients who are not proficient in the English language because these clients will find it difficult to comprehend what is being taught. To overcome this challenge, an RN can use an interpreter, use simple words and phrases and also use diagrams and demonstrations.

Age – Age has a huge impact on understanding and comprehension. To overcome this challenge, RNs should use teaching methods that are appropriate for each client's age.

Level of Literacy – The teaching methods an RN uses for a client who can read and write will be different from the methods used for a client with low literacy. To overcome this challenge, an RN should assess a client's literacy level. It is good to ask direct questions about the client's level of education.

Stressors – Stressors like pain, worry and anxiety are obstacles to effective learning. An RN should choose the appropriate time to teach. Teaching should only come after patients' basic physiological needs are met.

Health Beliefs – The cultural, religious and social beliefs a client has towards health will greatly impact his/her willingness to listen and learn. For example, a client may believe that vaccines cause autism in children. Another client may believe that traditional healers are more efficient than medical health workers, and so on. To overcome this challenge, the nurse must be aware of the origin of these health beliefs and address them by using reason and logic. In doing so, the nurse should use therapeutic communication techniques to prevent/minimize conflict.

Cognitive Function – Mental disorders, learning disorders and psychological disorders are just a few of the factors that can affect the cognition of a client. To overcome this challenge, RNs should use simple teaching methods. If cognitive function is severely affected, a guarantor can step in on the client's behalf.

Functional Limitation – Functional impairments of sight, sound and speech can affect the efficiency of learning. To overcome this challenge, RNs should use teaching methods that are best adapted to a client's abilities.

Nursing Research

Nursing research provides verifiable evidence that supports and improves nursing practices. This aspect of nursing education places a strong emphasis on the use of scientific evidence to explain nursing interventions. Nursing research can either be qualitative or quantitative.

Qualitative Nursing Research Method

This research method is used to explore and describe phenomena. The method uses flexible study designs, open-ended questions and unstructured and semi-structured methods to categorize responses to questions. The aim of this research method is to describe variation, describe and explain the relationship between two variables, describe individual experiences and describe group norms.

Types of Qualitative Research Models

Ethnographic Model – This is a very popular research model. The aim of this research model is to describe the cultural characteristics that drive a group. In nursing, ethnography is important in understanding a client's response to health care. This is important because a client's religious and cultural beliefs have a great impact on how someone receives, accepts and responds to medical care.

Phenomenological Model – This model uses surveys, questionnaires and interviews to describe how a participant experiences an event. This model is focused on how participants feel about an event. This model is important in helping nurses understand and improve nursing care delivery systems.

Grounded Theory Model – This model seeks to explain participants' behavior by using existing data to observe the actions of large numbers of subjects.

Case Study Model – This model is used to observe and theorize the actions of a single test subject. Unlike the grounded theory model that observes large numbers of subjects, the case study model uses a single subject, i.e., a person, family or city.

Historical Model – This model attempts to describe past events so as to understand present client patterns and anticipate future trends. This model uses a hypothetical idea to test for deviations.

Narrative Model – This model observes data over a long period of time. It studies subjects from a starting point and reviews their outcomes as they face obstacles and opportunities.

Quantitative Research Method

This research method is used to confirm a hypothesis. The method uses rigid study designs, close-ended questions and structured methods to categorize responses to questions. The aim of this research method is to quantify variation, anticipate causal relationships and describe characteristics of a population. Qualitative research uses numerical data.

Quantitative Research Models

Descriptive Model – This model aims to describe the current features of a variable and provide information about a variable. Usually the researcher begins without a hypothesis and develops one after collating the necessary data.

Correlational Model – In this model, the researcher attempts to use statistics to determine the relationship between two or more variables. This model does not study the cause and effect relationship between variables but describes the distribution of data.

Quasi-experimental Model – This is also known as the causal-comparative experimental model. In this model, the researcher attempts to describe the cause and effect relationships between variables. This model differs from a true experimental research model because an independent variable is not manipulated; instead, the researcher uses preexisting groups. Also, the effects of the independent variable on the dependent variable are measured.

Experimental Research Model – This model is also called true experimental research. The researcher uses scientific methods to establish the cause and effect relationships between variables.

In this model, the independent variable is identified and manipulated to determine its effect on the dependent variable. Subjects are randomly assigned to groups.

Importance of Nursing Research

1. **Evidence-Based Practice** – Nursing research provides scientific and verified information necessary for improving evidence-based practice. This is because the outcomes of nursing research are used to improve clinical decisions and clinical care. Peer-reviewed data is valid, reliable and relevant data that guides the best nursing practices.

2. **Information Literacy** – Scholarly articles help nurses to interpret data, process information, critique results and compare the outcome of different

studies. These abilities help an RN to use this information to provide evidence-based care.

3. **Professional Accountability** – Publishing a scholarly article requires professional accountability and reliance. Peer-reviewed articles are usually assessed for their originality, validity, reliability and relevance. As a result, RNs go through a rigorous process of critical thinking, writing, proofreading and fact-checking to create a work that meets the required standard.

4. **Problem Solving** – Nursing research improves the problem-solving skills of an RN. This is because research is based on the ability to identify, describe or quantify phenomena that involve problems unique to nursing care practices. For example, an RN who decides to do research on pediatric care will identify the phenomenon in pediatric care and decide on the best way to describe it, either by using quantitative or qualitative research methods.

5. **Teaching** – Nursing research improves the teaching skills of an RN. This is because nursing research enhances the ability of a nurse to use problem-solving, critical thinking, clinical judgment, communication and organization.

Culture and Spirituality

As society becomes more interconnected, nurses and health-care workers need to demonstrate cultural competence. Cultural competence is an ability to be self-aware while also maintaining awareness of a client's cultural identity. Cultural competence encourages self-awareness, acceptance, knowledge and acceptance of others.

Culturally competent nurses are able to provide individualized care to a diverse set of clients. A culturally competent nurse can be trusted by clients. This trust forms the basis of nurse-client interactions and compliance. It reduces hospital stays.

Barriers to Cultural Competence

Barriers to cultural competence include provider barriers and system barriers. Provider barriers are individual barriers that may be experienced by a healthcare worker, while system barriers are seen in organizations whose policies aren't designed to nurture cultural diversity. Provider barriers include language, bias, misinformation and ignorance. System barriers include policies, laws and administration that favor one cultural identity above others. In 2016, JoAnn Zerwekh developed a mnemonic, "CULTURE," for assessing cultural competence:

1. **C**onsider your own cultural bias and how it affects your nursing care.
2. **U**nderstand the need to recognize cultural implications in planning and implementing nursing care.
3. **L**earn how to use cultural assessment tools.
4. **T**reat patients with dignity and respect.
5. **U**se sensitivity in providing culturally competent care.
6. **R**ecognize opportunities to provide specific, culturally based nursing care.
7. **E**valuate your own previous encounters with patients from other cultures and backgrounds.

Spirituality

People tend to confuse religion with spirituality, even when these are two separate terms. Religion is an institution, while spirituality is individualized. Religion is founded on dogma and doctrine, while spirituality is based on individual experiences and perceptions. Because there is no clear-cut definition of spirituality, an RN can find it difficult to provide spiritual nursing care.

One definition of spiritual nursing care is "an intuitive, interpersonal, altruistic and integrative expression that is contingent upon the nurse's awareness of the transcendent dimension of life but that reflects the patient's reality" (Sawatzky and Pesut, 2005, p. 23). An RN should be aware of a client's spiritual needs and create spiritual interventions as appropriate.

Identifying Spiritual Needs

There are different methods a nurse can use to identify the spiritual needs of a client. They include:

Communicate with the Client and Family Members – It is important that the nurse know the client's religious beliefs before providing spiritual care. Family members can also offer insight into the client's beliefs.

Assess the Health Status of the Patient – It is a known fact that terminally ill and end-of-life patients show a need for spiritual care. In this phase, clients and their family members are concerned with the concept of the afterlife.

Close Observation – By observing a client's environment, demeanor and body language, a nurse can identify a need for spiritual care. For example, a Catholic client may hang a rosary on a drawer, or a Muslim client may have prayer beads and a Qur'an. A Pentecostal Christian may have a Bible.

Direct Expression – A client can directly express his need for spiritual care by asking for a Bible or a holy scripture or a comfortable position to pray, for example.

Forms of Spiritual Interventions

Spiritual interventions can be religious and non-religious. Religious interventions include prayer, meditation, scripture reading, pastoral care, chants, music and so on. Non-religious interventions include allowing longer visits from family members, active listening, hand-holding and deliberate silence.

Chapter 3: Content Overview

Client Needs

The Client Needs model is used for assessment because it has a universal structure for assessing entry-level nursing actions. Also, this framework is patient-centered in all settings of nursing care.

There are four major Client Needs categories, with two of the four categories divided into subcategories. They are:

1. Safe and Effective Care Environment

A. Management of Care – 17% to 23%

B. Safety and Infection Control – 9% to 15%

2. Health Promotion and Maintenance

3. Psychosocial Integrity

4. Physiological Integrity

A. Basic Care and Comfort – 6% to 12%

B. Pharmacological and Parenteral Therapies – 12% to 18%

C. Reduction of Risk Potential – 9% to 15%

D. Physiological Adaptation – 11% to 17%

Note that the percentages describe the number of test questions allotted to each Client Need.

1. Safe and Effective Care Management

This section is divided into two subsections: management of care and safety and infection control.

1A. Management of Care

Management of care makes up 17-23% of test questions assigned to each candidate. In this section, the candidate is expected to know the principles of nursing care that apply to advance directives, advocacy, informed consent, legal rights, assignment, delegation and supervision, case management, client rights, collaboration, concepts of management, confidentiality, continuity of care, establishing priorities, ethical practice, information technology, performance improvement, risk management and referrals.

Advance Directives

The candidate is assessed on the ability to:

1. Assess a client's understanding of advance directives – To assess a client's understanding of advance directives, an RN can ask the client direct questions to assess his/her perception, beliefs and knowledge.

2. Educate a client on available advance directive measures – If the client is uninformed, the RN must decide on the best learning method to use. Apart from educating the client, the RN is responsible for assessing and educating other members of the nursing team on the principles of advance directives.

3. Incorporate advance directives into the care plan – Advance directives are added to a client's management plan as early as possible. To do this, the RN reviews and confirms the advance directive status of the client from the onset of admission. The aim is to facilitate smooth and prompt delivery of management, especially in emergency cases.

Alternatives to Advance Directives

Advance directives are legal documents that direct and guide health-care decisions made for end-of-life clients. They afford clients the right and authority to decide on a care plan, even when clients are no longer competent to do so for themselves. Alternatives to advance directives include a living will, a DNR order, a physician order for life-sustaining treatment, a durable power of attorney and opting for organ donation.

1. Living will – A client uses a living will to state future health-care decisions when he/she is no longer able to make those choices on his own. The living will is usually used by terminally ill and end-of-life clients. This legal document outlines the conditions for when life will be prolonged or a natural death will be allowed to occur. It also states the conditions for certain treatments like dialysis, feeding, life support and others. A client can annul a living will at any time.

2. Durable power of attorney – Durable power of attorney is also known as medical power of attorney. This is a legal document in which a client names an agent to make all health-care decisions when the client is unable to do so. Before a client's durable power of attorney is accepted, the physician assesses whether the client is capable of making medical decisions. Durable power of attorney laws vary from state to state.

3. A physician order for life-sustaining treatment (POLST) – A POLST helps a client describe his/her preferences for health care. A POLST is different from an advance directive because a POLST is a form with specific options for a client to choose from. For example, a client can decide what care should be provided in an emergency. For example, a person can decide if he/she wants CPR, a ventilator or to be taken to the hospital. Unlike an advance directive

that must be signed by a physician, a POLST can be signed by paramedics and emergency medical technicians. POLST forms are only available in some states.

4. Do Not Resuscitate Orders (DNR) – A DNR order is used by clients who don't wish to be resuscitated when their heart fails. Some hospitals require clients to sign a new DNR order form each time they are admitted. A DNR is only used in hospitals.

Advocacy

In this subsection, candidates will be assessed on the ability to:

1. Discuss and respect treatment options chosen by a client – An RN advocates for clients by discussing treatment options without bias. This includes a discussion on the benefits and risks of the treatment, its principles, possible alternatives and information on those performing the procedures or carrying out the treatment plan.

2. Educate staff on advocacy – RNs educate other staff members on concepts like the function of the nursing care team as an advocate for clients' rights and autonomy and the available resources for acting as advocates.

3. Utilize advocacy resources – This involves collaboration with other professionals like social workers, clergy, home-care agencies, professional interpreters, etc.

Informed Consent

The candidate is assessed on the ability to:

1. Identify the recipient of informed consent – A recipient of informed consent must be an adult who is mentally competent and can comprehend the

implications of medical treatment. If the client is a minor or incompetent, consent can be obtained on his/her behalf. For example, consent can be obtained from a parent, legal guardian, a guarantor of a durable power of attorney and/or a legally appointed representative.

2. Describe the components of informed consent – Informed consent is permission granted for medical treatment after educating the client on the benefits and risks.

Consent can be implicit, explicit or implied. Components of informed consent include:

- The type of treatment or procedure
- The person who will perform the treatment
- The purpose of the treatment
- The expected outcome of the treatment
- The possible risks of the treatment
- The possible alternatives
- The benefits and risks of the available alternatives
- The client's right to refuse the treatment.

3. Verify that the client understands the principles of the care management plan – Before informed consent is obtained, the nurse must confirm that the client understands the principles of the management plan and procedures. The nurse should confirm this by asking direct questions to assess the client's grasp of the concepts explained.

Legal Rights

The candidate will be assessed on the ability to:

1. Identify legal issues affecting treatment – These issues typically revolve around informed consent, a client's right to refuse treatment, negligence, malpractice, licensure and others.

2. Educate client and staff on legal issues – The nurse must educate the client and other members of the staff on legal issues revolving around common law, civil law, criminal law, statutory law, administrative law and other legal concepts.

A. Common Law – This law is based on custom and judicial precedents. e.g., right to refuse treatment.

B. Constitutional Law – This law is included in the Constitution of the United States.

C. Statutory Law – This law is passed by a legislative body such as the US Congress.

D. Administrative Law – This is made up of rules and regulations that are enacted to support a statutory law. e.g., the administrative law enacted by the state nursing boards.

E. Criminal Law – This covers acts that are illegal, e.g., felony, fraud, theft, practicing without a license and practicing with an expired license.

F. Civil Law – This law covers disputes between people and infractions against the legal rights of individuals, e.g., negligence, malpractice, assault and battery.

3. Review existing policies and regulations – The nurse must be up to date on the existing policies that regulate the provision of health care.

4. Report client conditions – Conditions like abuse, neglect, gunshot wounds, assault and communicable diseases must be reported to the appropriate bodies.

5. Report unsafe health-care practices – Unsafe health-care practices used by both licensed and unlicensed health-care workers must be reported to the appropriate administrative bodies.

6. Care for the client according to the legal scope of nursing practice – Nurses must only provide care that is within their scope of practice. This is to prevent medico-legal issues.

Assignment, Delegation and Supervision

In this section, the candidate will be assessed on the ability to:

1. Identify tasks for delegation based on a client's needs – An RN must be skilled at matching the needs of the patient to the skill of the health personnel. This is important in providing client-centered care that is safe and efficient.

2. Assess the knowledge and skill of the personnel before delegating tasks – The RN must know the job description and scope of service of all health personnel. The RN can do this by looking up the state's scope of practice.

3. Communicate with other members of the team – RNs must communicate changes and significant findings to the doctors, supervising nurses and other members of the multidisciplinary team.

4. Evaluate delegated tasks – Nursing assistants and LPNs must relate the outcome of their delegated tasks to the RN.

5. Understand the five rights of delegation – The five rights of delegation include the right person, the right task, the right circumstances, the right direction and the right supervision.

6. Supervise care provided by nursing assistants and LPNs – The RN must be available to teach, monitor and supervise nursing care and interventions delegated to nursing assistants and LPNs.

Case Management

In this section, the candidate is assessed on his/her ability to:

1. Assess the client's need for medical resources – An RN is responsible for determining the medical equipment, materials and resources necessary to improve the client's health. Materials could include a CPAP machine, an oxygen ventilator, a suctioning machine and so on.

2. Explore available resources for maintaining a client's independence – This includes financial and human resources necessary for improving client outcomes. This resource should be cost-effective without compromising the quality of care given.

3. Plan individualized client-centered care – An RN is responsible for providing care that is tailored to meet the client's physical, physiological, sociological and social needs.

4. Educate clients on prevention methods and discharge procedures – A discharge plan is a continuum. A nurse is responsible for educating clients on the discharge procedures to the home, community or hospice center. Apart from that, nurses, along with other members of the health team, are involved in monitoring a client's discharge process in an outpatient setting.

5. Evaluating and updating the care plan – An RN is also responsible for updating the care plan, ensuring that it reflects the current status of the client.

Client Rights

In this section, the candidate is examined on the ability to:

1. Respect the client's right to refuse treatment – The Patient Self-Determination Act gives the client a right to decide on his/her management plan.

2. Discuss available treatment options – This is part of informed consent.

3. Educate the client and other staff on the rights and responsibilities of a client – An RN must take the time to educate the client on his/her rights. Other members of staff must also be educated.

4. Act as an advocate for the client's needs – An RN is an advocate for the rights and needs of the client.

Collaboration

In this section, the candidate is assessed on the knowledge and ability to:

1. Collaborate with other members of the health-care team – This function requires the use of interpersonal skills, critical thinking, clinical judgment and teamwork.

2. Communicate important information to other health disciplines – The RN must assess a client all throughout treatment and report significant findings to the appropriate health personnel.

3. Recognize the importance of collaboration and interdependence – An RN must recognize the importance of specialization in health care.

Concepts of Management

In this section, the candidate is assessed on the ability to:

1. Create nursing care plans to address client needs – An RN is responsible for interpreting data collected by LPNs, making diagnoses and implementing nursing care plans.
2. Evaluate management outcomes – The nurse is responsible for reassessing the client and evaluating outcomes of the care management plan.
3. Handle conflict amongst other members of the team – An RN is involved in administrative duties, which include overseeing the smooth functioning of the nursing team.

Confidentiality

In this section, the candidate will be assessed on the ability to:

1. Evaluate the client's understanding of confidentiality requirements – This includes assessing the client's knowledge of the Health Insurance Portability and Accountability Act (HIPAA).
2. Maintain the client's confidentiality – This involves making information available only to members of the management team. They include the client, the client's significant other and the health personnel involved in the management.
3. Intervene when there is a breach of privacy – A nurse must intervene when there is unauthorized access to medical records, a lack of confidentiality during shifts and others.

Continuity of Care

In this section, the candidate is assessed on the ability to:

1. Provide reports on assigned clients – Reports are usually evaluated at the end of each shift. These reports usually include the patient's name, the doctor's

name, date of admission, diagnosis, medical and nursing care plans, patient's physiological data and investigation results.

2. Document client's information – Documentation may include case notes, progress reports, vital sign charts, input and output forms and so on.

3. Perform procedures necessary to admit, transfer and discharge a client – RNs are involved in preparing medical records and documents for transferring, admitting and discharging clients.

Establishing Priorities

In this section, the candidate is assessed on the ability to:

1. Prioritize client care – This function requires skill in critical thinking and clinical judgment.

2. Evaluate nursing care plans of multiple patients – An RN is responsible for prioritizing multiple patients according to the urgency of their physiological needs. Examples of these needs include airway, breathing, circulation, excretion, food and so on.

3. Apply the principles of pathophysiology to prioritize clients – An RN must be able to apply the principles of pathophysiologic processes. This will help in prioritization and creation of action plans in emergency settings.

Ethical Practice – In this section, the candidate is assessed on the ability to:

1. Recognize and address ethical dilemmas – An RN must be skilled in the ethical decision-making process, which includes problem definition, data collection, data analysis, identification, selecting the best possible solution, performing the selected desired course of action and evaluating the results of the action.

2. Educate clients and staff on ethical issues affecting client care – An RN must educate clients on the ethical implications of their current management plan. Other members of the nursing team are also duly informed.
3. Uphold ethical principles in nursing practice – An RN should be guided by ethical principles of justice, beneficence, nonmaleficence, accountability, fidelity, autonomy and veracity.

Information Technology

In this section, the candidate is evaluated on his/her ability to:

1. Access and store data in online databases – RNs are required to input and retrieve data from different forms of electronic records.
2. Use information technology to improve client care – RNs must use information technology to access information for clients. Sources of information include online journals, PDF files and verified websites.

Performance Improvement and Risk Management

In this section, the candidate is assessed on his/her ability to identify performance improvement, engage in a process that enhances performance and assess the impact of performance on client care.

Referrals

In this section, the candidate is assessed on his/her ability to assess clients who are in need of specialized care, identify the documents required for a referral and recognize the value of timely referrals. RNs must also be equipped to identify resources for clients in an outpatient setting. These resources include social work services, group therapy, housing, emergency shelters, hospice centers and home centers.

1B. Safety and Infection Control

This section assesses the candidate's ability to protect the client and other health personnel from hazards. That comprises 9-15% of the section. Subsections include accident and incident prevention, emergency response plans, principles of ergonomics, handling hazardous and infectious materials, home safety, reporting incidents and irregular occurrences, safe use of equipment, security plans, observance of standard precautions and use of restraints and safety devices.

Accident and Incident Prevention

In this section, the candidate is assessed on the ability to:

1. Determine the client's knowledge of safety procedures – Staff members and their employers are assessed on their knowledge of workplace safety procedures. This assessment can be done by performing surveys and using questionnaires.

2. Examine clients for allergies and treat as indicated – This includes assessing a client for allergies to food, latex, dander, pollen, medications, contrast media and others. This assessment is performed by collecting data on previous medical histories.

3. Identify the factors that place clients at risk for accidents and injuries – A nurse must be able to identify factors like age, cognitive and physiological impairment, substance abuse, lifestyle choice and other factors that put clients at risk.

4. Identify impairments and disabilities that can hinder a client's safety – This includes an assessment of physical, physiological and cognitive deficits that increase a client's risk for injuries.

5. Teach clients methods to alert others – This involves the use of systems like bells, alarms and calls to alert people of impending danger. Drills should be done regularly to assess people's response to emergencies.
6. Follow seizure safety protocols for those at risk – Such protocols include the use of bars and rails to prevent falls, the use of mouthpieces to prevent tongue lacerations and correct positioning of the client to prevent aspiration. Also, clients with seizure disorders should be counseled to avoid activities like driving and climbing, to prevent the risk of injuries. Such clients should also be counseled to wear emergency tags and bracelets to alert others of their condition.
7. Identify clients when giving care – Identification of clients is the first step before beginning any medical intervention. This is done for medical and legal reasons.

Emergency Response Plans

In this section, the candidate is assessed on the ability to:

1. Prioritize client care – When caring for multiple clients in the emergency room, an RN must use critical thinking and clinical judgment to prioritize a client's needs according to the urgency of physiological needs. For example, a client with an acute hemorrhage should be prioritized over a client with a dislocated arm.
2. Determine whether a client is fit for discharge – An RN must assess whether clients are fit for discharge. Doing so reduces traffic, reduces the workload and reduces the risk of nosocomial infections.
3. Identifying nursing care protocol in disaster planning – RNs must follow specific rules in managing both internal and external disasters. For example,

the roles of all health workers should be clearly outlined in the management of disasters like fires, utility failures, bomb threats, radiation contamination and others.

4. Take part in drills – Nurses must take part in routine drills to assess and strengthen their response to emergencies.
5. Create an emergency response plan – An RN is involved in creating emergency response plans for both stable and unstable patients.

Principles of Ergonomics

In this section, the candidate is assessed on the ability to:

1. Use ergonomic principles in providing care – This involves educating clients on the proper use of assistive devices like walking canes, crutches and trolleys. Also, the nurse uses the principles of body mechanics in bending, lifting and moving objects and people.
2. Teach clients principles of proper body posture – An RN must educate clients on appropriate posture when walking, sitting and using assistive devices.
3. Evaluate a client's ability to use assistive devices like walking canes and crutches.

Handling Hazardous and Infectious Materials

In this section, the candidate is assessed on the ability to:

1. Identify various biohazards and infectious materials – This includes infectious plastic materials like urethral catheters, infusions and blood-transfusion sets. It also includes non-recyclable infectious materials like used cotton swabs, abdo packs, linens, placenta and tissues, sharps and needles, expired drugs and radioactive waste.

2. Know the principles of handling and disposing of biohazardous waste – Biohazardous waste must be disposed of in an appropriate waste container. For example, sharps are disposed of in the sharps container. Some facilities use color codes for waste disposal. For example, expired drugs and radioactive waste are disposed of in black waste containers. Infectious non-plastic materials are disposed of in yellow waste containers. Infectious plastic waste is disposed of in red containers.

3. Follow safety guidelines concerning internal radiation therapy – Some of these safety guidelines include placing the client in a private room before, during, and after radiotherapy, educating the client on the benefits and risks of radiotherapy and minimizing visiting time after radiotherapy.

Home Safety

In this section, the candidate is assessed on the ability to:

1. Evaluate clients who need home and environment modifications – Clients with physical, physiologic and cognitive impairment will benefit from environment modification to reduce the risk of home accidents. For example, an elderly client with Parkinson's will benefit from improved lighting in the hallways, with rails and banisters installed on staircases.

2. Incorporate pathophysiology into home-safety principles – During an assessment, an RN must use the features of the client's pathophysiology to create safety principles that are tailored to the client's needs. For example, a visually impaired client will benefit from an environment that is free from hazards like throw rugs and electrical cords.

3. Educate the client on home safety rules – Apart from assessing the environment and making necessary interventions to avoid home accidents,

the nurse must educate clients on the benefits of home safety rules and principles.

4. Encourage the client to wear protective equipment when using hazardous materials – An RN's work isn't restricted to just a hospital setting. An RN can educate industrial workers on the importance of wearing the right equipment for protection. For example, iron welders should wear the right type of eye goggles, gloves and earphones to prevent physical hazards caused by light, sound and heat.

5. Assess the client's environment for fire and environmental hazards – An RN must assess a client's environment for smoke alarms, frayed electrical cords, food safety, fire extinguishers, handrails and carbon monoxide alarms.

Reporting Incidents and Irregular Occurrences

In this section, the candidate is assessed on the ability to:

1. Identify events that require reporting of incidents and irregular occurrences – An RN must be familiar with a health facility's protocols and policies on reporting irregular occurrences.

2. Document practice errors – All medical errors should be documented for medical and legal reasons. The nurse must also record the interventions made to correct these errors and the client's response to the interventions.

Safe Use of Equipment

In this section, the candidate is assessed on the ability to:

1. Inspect equipment and eliminate hazards – An RN must examine any equipment that is a potential safety hazard. This includes frayed cords, missing parts, loose parts and evidence of malfunctions.

2. Educate clients on the proper use of equipment – An RN must educate clients on the medical equipment each client requires, especially when this equipment will be used for home care. For example, a client should be educated on the proper use of an oxygen tank to prevent the risk of fire.
3. Assess and remove malfunctioning equipment from the area – An RN must ensure that any malfunctioning equipment is removed, replaced and/or sent to be repaired.

Security Plan

In this section, the candidate is assessed on the ability to:

1. Engage in the institution's security plan – Health-care facilities mandate personnel to prepare for emergencies and disasters. To do this, they encourage personnel to perform drills and review a facility's protocol on security and emergencies.
2. Use principles of triage and evacuation procedures – An RN must be familiar with the principles of the evacuation of clients in case of emergencies. For example, ambulatory clients are the first to be discharged, followed by stable patients. Unstable clients are not discharged except in extreme circumstances.
3. Use clinical judgment and critical thinking to create security plans – An RN must use clinical and critical thinking to participate in security plans and perform security drills.

Observance of Standard Precautions

In this section, the candidate is assessed on the ability to:

1. Know the various routes of transmission of communicable diseases – Communicable disease can be transmitted through air, by contact or by vectors. A nurse must have knowledge of the different routes of transmission of communicable disease and the different isolation protocols.
2. Apply principles of infection control – These principles include the use of personal protective equipment, handwashing and the use of various protocols to reduce airborne, droplet and contact transmission of diseases.
3. Set up a sterile field – An RN must set up sterile fields by following the basic rules of asepsis. For example, sterile items are used in a sterile field. The sterile field must be kept dry and moisture-free. Sterile gowns and gloves should always be worn in a sterile field. Nurses should avoid coughing, sneezing or leaning over a sterile field, etc.
4. Educate the client and team members on principles of infection control – An RN must assess each client's knowledge of infection control measures and then decide the most effective teaching method to educate each client.
5. Supervise aseptic techniques used by LPNs and nursing assistants – An RN is responsible for the direct supervision of nursing assistants and LPNs as they carry out aseptic procedures. A nurse must determine whether aseptic technique is performed correctly and ensure that measures for infection control are followed.
6. Use the proper guidelines for immunocompromised clients – Immunocompromised clients are at risk of contracting diseases transmitted through respiratory, droplet or contact routes. To minimize the risk of infection, protective precautions must be taken. For example, immunocompromised clients should always be kept in rooms with positive pressure.

Infection Control and Prevention

Standard Precaution

This infection control protocol is used to prevent the transmission of diseases that can be spread by contact with infectious blood, body fluids, mucous membranes and broken skin. This protocol is used for all clients, regardless of whether they are infectious or not. They include:

Hand Hygiene – This practice involves thorough and strict handwashing. Handwashing is done with plain or antibacterial soap or a hand sanitizer that contains at least 60% alcohol. Hand hygiene should be observed:

- Before and after contact with a client
- Immediately after handling body fluids
- After touching non-intact skin and mucous membranes
- Immediately after removing gloves
- Before moving from a contaminated to a decontaminated area
- After coming in contact with a client's environment
- After using medical equipment
- After using the restroom
- Before eating
- After coughing and sneezing

Personal Protective Equipment – Components of PPE include gloves, gowns, masks, respirators and eye goggles. These materials are used to protect the wearer from pathogens that can come in contact with skin, clothing, the respiratory tract and mucous membranes. The type of PPE worn depends on the transmission of contact from a client to a health worker. Gloves are used to protect health workers' hands from infectious body fluids, infectious mucus membranes and broken skin.

Surgical masks are used to protect health workers' nasal and oral mucosa from infectious pathogens. Eye goggles are worn to protect the eyes from infectious blood splashes and other body fluids. Gowns are worn to protect against pathogens spread via direct and indirect contact.

Prevention of Sharps Injuries – This protocol protects the client from bloodborne pathogens.

1. Activate safety devices on needles and other sharps immediately after use.
2. Discard used needles immediately after use. Do not recap, bend, cut or manipulate the needle from the syringe.
3. Discard used needles and sharps in a leak-proof, puncture-resistant sharps container.
4. Discard the sharps container when it is two-thirds full.

Cleaning and Disinfection – This protocol includes all the cleaning precautions taken to disinfect materials and surfaces.

1. Surfaces must be cleaned of organic matter and dirt before being disinfected.
2. Disinfectants must be used according to the susceptibility of the pathogen. For example, norovirus and *Clostridium difficile* are not inactivated by routine disinfectants. Instead, a bleach solution that is diluted in parts must be used.

Respiratory Hygiene – This protocol is used to avoid the transmission of respiratory secretions.

1. Cover the nose and mouth with a tissue when coughing or sneezing.
2. Use the crook of the elbow to contain droplets if a tissue is not available.

3. Wash your hands immediately after contact with respiratory droplets.
4. Encourage clients with respiratory disease to wear surgical masks.
5. Encourage clients to sit at least three feet apart in waiting rooms.
6. Supply waiting rooms with tissues, hand sanitizer, surgical masks, wastebaskets and handwashing sinks.

Waste Disposal – This protocol is used for the safe disposal of hospital waste and other biohazards.

1. Dispose of used sharps in the sharps container.
2. Disposable and infectious non-sharp items must be disposed of in leak-proof and puncture-resistant biohazard bags.
3. Radioactive waste must be disposed of in the appropriate container.

Safe Injection Practices – This protocol is used to protect health workers from bloodborne pathogens like hepatitis B and C.

1. Use a new needle and syringe for every IV medication.
2. Use a new needle and syringe for every intravenous access.

Transmission-Based Precaution

There are three types of transmission-based precautions: contact precaution, droplet precaution and airborne precaution.

Contact Precaution – This is used to prevent the transmission of pathogens that are spread by direct and indirect contact. Some of these pathogens include norovirus, rotavirus and parasitic infections like lice and scabies.

1. Wear gloves and gowns when in contact with the client and surfaces and objects within the client's environment.

2. Reusable items should be disinfected before being removed from the environment.
3. Disposable materials should be discarded at the point of use.
4. Observe standard protocol.

Droplet Precaution – This is used to prevent pathogens that are transmitted by droplets. Examples are influenza, meningococcal disease, streptococcus and others. Precautionary measures include:

1. Wear a surgical mask when within three feet of the infected individual.
2. Observe standard protocol.

Airborne Precaution – This is used to prevent the transmission of pathogens that are spread by fine particles dispersed by air currents. Examples are measles, SARS and tuberculosis.

1. Wear a certified and fit-tested N95 respirator just before entry into a shared space with the individual. Discard the respirator immediately after exiting the area.
2. Observe all standard protocols.
3. It is important to note that some diseases require the observation of more than one protocol. For example, to prevent the transmission of SARS, health workers should observe contact, droplet and airborne precaution.

Use of Restraints and Safety Devices

In this section, the candidate is expected to:

1. Know the indications of different restraining devices – RNs must determine whether restraints should be used on a client and, if restraints are needed,

which types are best. Restraints can be physical or chemical. Physical restraints include vests, padded wrist restraints, arm and leg restraints and side rails. Chemical restraints are drugs given to tranquilize agitated clients, not necessarily for therapeutic outcomes. For example, benzodiazepines are given intravenously to restrain manic clients.

2. Follow the guidelines and principles for each restraining device – An RN must follow guidelines to prevent complications when using restraints. Some of these guidelines include the evaluation of alternative methods to restraints, monitoring the client throughout the use of the restraints and using the least restrictive restraints possible.

3. Monitor the client's response to a restraining device – An RN must observe and document a client's physiological and emotional response to a restraint. Physiological data to be monitored includes the client's temperature, blood pressure and respiration. The nurse should also check for bruises, pallor and any signs of physical injury. Emotional states such as fear, anger and agitation must be assessed. The nurse should also monitor the client's cognitive state for signs of confusion and disorientation.

4. Evaluate the appropriateness of restraints used – Restraints should be used for the shortest time possible. To make this possible, the nurse must monitor the client's response to the use of the restraints. Adjustments can then be made as needed, either by removing the restraints or by using a less restrictive restraint. Alternative methods can also be employed. For example, an agitated client can be removed from the source of the agitation.

5. Provide care to restrained clients – Apart from monitoring the client's response to the use of restraints, a nurse must also provide care which includes turning and repositioning the client, providing skin care in the event

of bruises and injuries and providing physiological needs like food, hydration and assistance with elimination of waste.

Chapter 4: Health Promotion and Maintenance

This section makes up about 6-12% of the NCLEX-RN test questions. In this section, the candidate is assessed on his/her knowledge of growth and development, primary, secondary and tertiary prevention methods of disease.

Test sections include but are not limited to the aging process, health screening, ante/intra/postpartum care, developmental stages, health promotion, high-risk behavior, lifestyle choices, self-care and techniques of physical assessment.

Aging Process

In this section, the candidate is assessed on the ability to:

1. Assess clients' attitudes and beliefs towards age-related changes – These beliefs are associated with changes in body size and distribution of fat content, as seen in pregnant women. It also includes reproductive changes in teenagers and senile changes in the elderly, such as fecal and urinary incontinence, psychosocial and psychomotor changes and so on.

2. Provide care and health education for children 0-2 years old – An RN must provide care and health education on developmental milestones, hygiene, feeding and disease prevention.

3. Provide care and health education for clients 3-17 years old – An RN must provide care and health education on most primary prevention methods and educate clients and their parents on developmental changes.

4. Provide care and health education for clients 18-64 years old – Health education includes but is not limited to reproductive health education, mental health education, nutrition and personal and environmental hygiene.

5. Provide care and health education for clients 65-85 years old – Care provided to geriatric clients includes but is not limited to nursing care to make daily activities of feeding, dressing and bathing comfortable; psychological support for both the clients and the caregivers and drugs, food and exercise.

Ante/Intra/Postpartum and Newborn Care

In this section, the candidate is assessed on the ability to:

1. Assess a client's psychosocial response to pregnancy – This includes evaluating the factors that can influence a client's psychosocial response. Factors include age, socioeconomic status, marital status, culture and religious beliefs.

2. Evaluate symptoms of postpartum complications – These complications include but are not limited to postpartum hemorrhage, postpartum eclampsia, postpartum sepsis and postpartum depression.

3. Recognize cultural differences in childbearing – There are various cultural practices that affect childbearing. The nurse must pay close attention to clients from different ethnic backgrounds. Also, the nurse must ask direct questions to evaluate the client's cultural beliefs.

4. Calculate expected dates of delivery – The expected date of delivery is calculated from the client's last menstrual period. Early ultrasound scans are used as confirmation and also for calculating the expected delivery dates for women who can't recall their last menstrual period.

5. Educate new mothers on newborn care – New mothers are educated on newborn care which includes:

A. Eye care – Application of eye ointments containing erythromycin and chloramphenicol. These antibiotics are needed for prophylactic treatment of chlamydia and gonorrhea infections.

B. Cord care – The umbilical cord must be kept dry at all times. To do this, mothers are encouraged to give their babies sponge baths until the cord falls off.

C. Warmth – Newborns must be kept warm at all times to prevent hypothermia and pneumonia.

D. Food – Breast milk is the preferred milk of choice for infants. Mothers should be encouraged to breastfeed their babies exclusively for six months. After that, complementary feeds may be commenced. Mothers should be encouraged to breastfeed their babies until they are two years old.

E. Immunization – Vaccines like Hepatitis, OPV, DPT and IPV must be given in the first month of life.

6. Provide prenatal care and education – Prenatal care includes supplementation of necessary micronutrients like folic acid and iron. Prenatal screening should be used to assess the risk of congenital abnormalities. These risk factors include diabetes mellitus, current drug use, exposure to radiation, screening and sexually transmitted infections.

7. Provide postpartum care and education – This includes education on diet, nutrition, breastfeeding, emotional support, management of postpartum complications and education on family planning options and contraceptives.

8. Assess the client's ability to care for a newborn – New mothers should be evaluated on their ability to provide cord care, breastfeed and maintain

personal hygiene. They should also be evaluated on their knowledge of existing vaccinations.

Types of Immunity

1. Natural Active Immunity – This kind of immunity is created by the immune system when it is exposed to diseases. For example, a client who is exposed to the varicella zoster virus will develop antibodies. These antibodies have immunologic memory that will recognize the varicella zoster's antigen in the future and can then quickly neutralize it.

2. Natural Passive Immunity – This immunity is conferred by the transmission of antibodies from another person. For example, a mother transmits antibodies to her infant through breast milk. Breast milk is rich in IgA, IgG and IgM antibodies. IgA antibodies protect infants from common respiratory and gastrointestinal infections.

3. Artificial Active Immunity – This immunity is conferred when a client is exposed to artificially introduced antigens. For example, during vaccination, a client is injected with live-attenuated bacteria like pertussis, or toxoids like diphtheria and tetanus. These vaccines stimulate the client's immune system to produce antibodies and memory cells that can mount an immune response when it is re-exposed to these antigens in the future.

4. Artificial Passive Immunity – This immunity is conferred when immunoglobulins are artificially introduced into a client's body. For example, the human tetanus immunoglobulin is given to clients who are either at risk of having tetanus or who have tetanus.

Developmental Stages

In this section, the candidate is assessed on the ability to:

1. Evaluate expected physical, cognitive and psychosocial stages of development – These include the diverse social and motor developmental milestones for each age group.
2. Recognize body image changes associated with development and aging – These include senile changes in psychomotor and psychological functions.
3. Recognize the role of family members and structure – The nurse must assess the quality of support provided by family members and caregivers, whether the client is living alone, in a home center or with a family member.
4. Recognize deviations from normal developmental milestones – The nurse must be alert to red flags like delayed or absent developmental milestones.
5. Provide assistance for adjusting to developmental processes – Assistance can include supplying assistive devices, educating patients on comfortable bed positions and assisting with feeding, dressing and bathing.
6. Educate clients and staff on developmental changes and their impact – Clients and staff must be educated on the expected psychomotor and psychological changes in each developmental stage.

Developmental Stages

There are four key stages of growth and human development. They include infancy (birth to two years old), early childhood (three to eight years old), middle childhood (nine to eleven years old) and adolescence (twelve to eighteen years old).

Each stage has unique milestones which must be used by nurses and other health workers to assess a client's growth and development.

1. Infancy (birth to 2 years old)

Infancy is the stage where the baby grows rapidly after birth. Growth during infancy is said to be even faster than growth during adolescence. By the end of the first year, a baby will have doubled in length and tripled its weight.

An infant is called a newborn in the first 30 days of its life. A newborn has a slightly disproportionate head, short limbs and a protruding belly. A newborn sleeps for about 18 hours a day and feeds exclusively on breast milk until about six months. At six months, an infant starts crawling, can sit without support and begins learning to crawl. Also, the first set of milk teeth erupt. These teeth continue to erupt until about three years of age.

By 12 months, an infant begins saying its first words and can stand and walk with or without support. Although breast milk is supplemented with other meals by six months, infants should be breastfed until at least two years.

2. Early Childhood (3-8 years)

The early childhood stage includes toddlers. "Toddler" is used to describe a child who is learning to walk. This child is usually one to three years old. Apart from walking, at this stage, toddlers also develop other motor skills. By the end of their third year, toddlers can walk up the stairs, run and climb on chairs. They can scribble with a crayon, feed and dress themselves with help. They also develop verbal skills like speaking in simple sentences and phrases. By age five, children can recognize letters and words, carry on conversations and can use a pencil to trace letters and shapes. They may also be able to kick a ball and swing a bat.

3. Middle Childhood (9-11 years)

At this stage, children transition from home to school. Also, children interact with their peers and form friendships. Most children at this stage start losing their milk teeth and begin to grow permanent teeth. Children reach a growth spurt in adolescence.

4. Adolescence (12-18 years)

This stage marks the beginning of puberty and adulthood. Adolescence is a time of mental, emotional and social changes. During this stage, teenagers become able to think abstractly, try to establish an identity and seek independence. At this stage, they may challenge authority and endure peer pressure. Teenagers want to spend more time with their peers compared to other developmental stages. Teens may also experience mood swings as they learn to manage their emotions.

Health Promotion

In this section, the candidate is assessed on the ability to:

1. Identify risk factors for diseases – These risk factors can be modifiable risk factors like diet, sedentary lifestyle, alcohol consumption, cigarette use, substance abuse and others. Non-modifiable risk factors include age, sex, ethnicity and genetics.

2. Educate clients and communities on health risks – An RN must educate clients on the impact of modifiable and non-modifiable risk factors on health and disease progression.

3. Identify barriers to efficient learning – These barriers include literacy, socioeconomic status, cultural beliefs, physiological, psychological and cognitive impairments.

4. Educate the client on primary prevention methods – These methods can be general methods like handwashing and vaccination, or specific methods used to prevent both communicable and non-communicable disease.
5. Incorporate complementary therapies into health promotion activities – Some of these complementary activities include physiotherapy, group therapy and support groups.
6. Provide follow-up for clients – These follow-up visits include both clinic and home visits.
7. Organize community-based care – An RN may provide health education and care at the community level, teaching public health topics like vaccination, handwashing and food and water hygiene.

Health Screening

In this section, the candidate is assessed on the ability to:

1. Apply principles of pathophysiology to health screening – These include principles like inflammation, metabolic derangement, hemolysis and degeneration.
2. Assess risk factors linked to ethnicity – Ethnicity is implicated in certain non-communicable diseases like hypertension, certain cancers, autoimmune diseases and metabolic diseases.
3. Perform health and risk assessments – This is done by obtaining data from the client's medical history.
4. Perform targeted screening – Targeted screening is done to identify particular risk factors in specified at-risk groups. Examples of targeted

screening include PSA screening for males 55 years and above, breast mammography for females, cervical cancer screening for females, blood glucose screening for adults, blood pressure measurement for adults and STI screening for sexually active clients.

5. Use appropriate interviewing techniques to gather clinical data – These include the use of the various therapeutic communication techniques to encourage trust.

High-Risk Behavior

In this section, the candidate is assessed on the ability to:

1. Identify lifestyle practices that put a client's health at risk – These lifestyle practices are modifiable risk factors that make clients vulnerable to certain communicable and non-communicable diseases. For example, smoking is a high-risk behavior that puts a client at risk for lung cancer and chronic obstructive pulmonary disease. A sedentary lifestyle puts a client at risk for metabolic derangement of glucose, fat and protein, cardiovascular diseases and cancer.
2. Educate clients on the prevention and management of high-risk behaviors – These are primary prevention methods that protect clients from exposure to these diseases. These prevention methods include lifestyle modification and early screening.

Lifestyle Choice

In this section, the candidate is assessed on the ability to:

1. Evaluate a client's attitudes to sexuality and sexual health – This includes evaluation of factors like religious and cultural beliefs, socioeconomic status, age, sex, substance abuse, alcoholism and psychological disorders.

2. Evaluate a client's need for contraception – Factors that influence the use of contraception include health education, religion, cultural values, ages, sex, socioeconomic status and marital status.

3. Identify contraindications to all forms of contraceptives – A client's physiological data must be collected and assessed before choosing a contraceptive method. Examples of contraindications to using contraceptives include:

COCP – Thromboembolic disorders, coronary artery disease, breast carcinoma, liver tumors, suspected pregnancy, diabetes, hypertension, gallbladder disease and hyperlipidemia.

Progesterone contraceptives – Breast cancer, cervical cancer and suspected pregnancy.

IUCD – History of ectopic pregnancy, pelvic inflammatory disease and multiple sexual partners.

4. Educate the client on sexual health – Clients must be educated on the impact of sexual activity on reproductive health, types of STIs, routes of infection, the complications of STIs and available methods for preventing STIs. Also, post- and pre-menopausal clients should be counseled on available options to improve their sexual health.

5. Assess the client's alternative medicine practices – These practices include the use of supplements, hot and cold compresses, meditation and visualization, hypnosis, acupuncture, yoga, music therapy, etc.

Self-Care

In this section, the candidate is assessed on the ability to:

1. Evaluate a client's ability to manage care in the home – Family support, psychological and physiological impairments, co-morbidities, literacy and socioeconomic status are factors that should be considered when assessing a client's ability to care for himself/herself at home.

2. Collaborate with primary caregivers to meet goals – Primary caregivers are key players in promoting self-care in a patient. Support, encouragement and health education are a few ways an RN can collaborate with a primary caregiver in achieving this goal.

3. Identify a client's self-care needs before creating a care plan – Before creating a care plan, a nurse should assess the needs of a client and prioritize them according to urgency. For example, physiological needs like food, water, airway and breathing should be prioritized above social needs like support and belonging.

Techniques of Physical Assessment

In this section, the candidate is assessed on the ability to:

1. Apply the principles of nursing procedures to physical assessment – Physical assessment includes a general examination of the client and systemic examination of all the body systems. In a general examination, the client is inspected from head to toe for features like obesity, weight loss, jaundice,

pallor, cyanosis, finger clubbing, pedal edema and so on. Vital signs like temperature, respiration, pulse and blood pressure are measured. A systemic examination includes palpation, percussion and auscultation of organs.

2. Choose the appropriate physical assessment equipment and techniques – The appropriate equipment must be used with respect to the size and age of the client. For example, a bassinet should be used to weigh infants, while weighing scales are used to weigh older children. Also, the size of cuffs used for blood pressure measurement is important, to avoid erroneous readings. For example, a small cuff can produce a high blood pressure reading, while a largc cuff can produce a low blood pressure measurement.

3. Perform a comprehensive health assessment – A detailed health assessment is done for all the body systems. This includes health assessments for the neurological, cardiovascular, respiratory, gastrointestinal, renal, reproductive and musculoskeletal systems.

Chapter 5: Psychosocial Integrity

This section makes up about 6-12% of the overall test. In this section, the candidate is assessed on the ability to manage clients with mental illness and provide emotional and mental support for distressed clients. Subsections include abuse and neglect, behavioral interventions, coping mechanisms, crisis intervention, cultural awareness, end-of-life care, family dynamics, grief and loss, mental health concepts, religious and spiritual influences on health, sensory/perceptual alterations, stress management, substance use, support systems, therapeutic communication and therapeutic environments.

Abuse and Neglect

In this section, the candidate is assessed on the ability to:

1. Assess and identify an abused client and commence appropriate intervention – This includes observation of verbal and nonverbal cues given by an abused client. After that, prompt intervention should be provided based on the priority of needs. For example, security and safety are provided first for vulnerable victims.

2. Identify risk factors for different types of abuse – This includes the various risk factors for child abuse, elder abuse and domestic abuse. Risk factors can include but are not limited to family dynamics, substance abuse, psychiatric disorders, socioeconomic status and age and sex of the victim.

3. Initiate interventions for victims of abuse – These interventions are given based on a priority of needs. Examples of intervention include providing a safe and secure environment, treating physical injuries, providing psychotherapy and counseling.

4. Counsel victims of abuse on coping mechanisms – These coping mechanisms are taught and practiced in group and support therapies.

5. Provide a safe environment for an abused client – Abused clients need a safe and secure environment away from the perpetrators of abuse.

6. Assess a client's response to interventions – Nursing care interventions must be evaluated and readjusted according to a client's current needs.

Behavioral Interventions

In this section, the candidate is assessed on the ability to:

1. Assess a client's mental state, behavior and response to inappropriate behavior – Mental states such as level of consciousness, orientation, mood, affect and appearance must be assessed. Inappropriate behavior like aggression, depression and mania should be identified, and appropriate interventions must be taken.

2. Help orient the client in reality – Clients with disorientation need assistance in orienting themselves in reality. Interventions include the use of therapeutic communication techniques, reminders, calendars and clocks.

3. Encourage the client to participate in group sessions – Clients with psychiatric disorders should be encouraged to participate in group sessions to encourage support, sharing and self-expression.

4. Initiate behavioral management techniques – This involves the use of stress and relaxation techniques, exercise, complementary therapies and socialization.

5. Evaluate the client's response to care – Nursing care plans for clients with psychiatric disorders should be assessed and readjusted to reflect current needs.

6. Assist the client in reducing anxiety – This involves the use of relaxation techniques like deep breathing exercises, meditation and mindfulness and group therapy.

Coping Mechanisms

In this section, the candidate is assessed on the ability to:

1. Evaluate available support systems and resources – Clients should be educated on coping mechanisms such as problem-solving skills, relaxation techniques and therapeutic communication techniques.

2. Assess the client's ability to adapt to role changes – Clients may find it difficult to adjust to dependent roles. It is more difficult for clients to adjust if the roles are permanent.

3. Evaluate the client's response to the diagnosis of mental illness – Such responses can be dependent on certain factors like religious and cultural beliefs, family dynamics, age and level of health education.

4. Assist the client in coping with changes – Assistance can be in the form of therapeutic communication techniques, support groups and family therapy.

5. Assist the client with altered body image – Altered body image can occur in clients involved in fire incidents, disasters, trauma and car accidents.

6. Evaluate the use of defense mechanisms by a client – Some of these defense mechanisms include regression, sublimation, rationalization, intellectualization and projection, amongst others.

Defense Mechanisms

These are subconscious mechanisms used to protect the ego from intense feelings and stress. Unlike coping mechanisms, defense mechanisms are subconscious and can be maladaptive. Defense mechanisms were first described by Austrian psychiatrist Sigmund Freud.

1. Displacement – In this mechanism, the client redirects his negative feelings from the intended recipient to a neutral substitute. For example, a client who is upset with his boss at work may come home and take his anger out on his wife.

2. Suppression – In this mechanism, a client consciously forgets painful and unpleasant thoughts and experiences. This is common in rape victims who attempt to suppress the event and refuse to report to the authorities.

3. Sublimation – In this mechanism, the client attempts to deal with unpleasant experiences by placing them in a pleasant context.

4. Denial – In this mechanism, a client refuses to admit to a painful reality. This is usually seen in terminally ill clients.

5. Intellectualization – In this mechanism, a client attempts to reason an unpleasant experience rather than react to it.

6. Introjection – In this mechanism, the client subconsciously absorbs specific traits into the ego. For example, a physically abused child may absorb the violence of her perpetrator.

7. Projection – In this mechanism, the client blames others for his/her feelings and actions. For example, an alcoholic might blame an alcoholic father for his/her own drinking problem.

8. Reaction Formation – In this mechanism, a client subconsciously represses reactions to painful and unpleasant experiences and replaces these reactions with opposite responses. For example, an abused wife who feels angry with her abusive husband may remain loyal to him.

9. Regression – In this mechanism, a client retreats to an earlier developmental stage. This mechanism is commonly used by small children who find it difficult to cope with the birth of a new sibling.

Crisis Intervention

The candidate is evaluated on the ability to:

1. Assess the potential for violence in a client – This is done by assessing verbal and nonverbal cues and psychiatric history.

2. Identify the client in crisis – This includes assessing clients at risk of suicide or self-injury.

3. Use techniques in crisis intervention – Some of these techniques include the use of positive reinforcements, relaxation techniques, compliance with drugs and educating the client on the importance of care plans.

4. Apply the principles of psychopathology to crisis interventions – These principles help an RN plan and prioritize nursing interventions.

Cultural Awareness

The candidate is assessed on the ability to:

1. Recognize the impact of a client's culture and ethnicity on care plans – This includes identifying the client's individual beliefs on mental health and

wellness. A nurse must be accepting of diversity in cultural beliefs and have an open mind when providing nursing care.

2. Recognize cultural issues that impact a client's acceptance of psychiatric disease – For example, a client might believe that a psychiatric disorder is the result of a spell, jinx or supernatural activity.

3. Incorporate a client's cultural practices and beliefs when planning care – As long as these practices do not interfere with the quality of care provided, a nurse can incorporate the client's cultural practices as alternative therapies.

4. Use appropriate interpreters to facilitate efficient learning – A nurse should use interpreters for clients who are not proficient in English.

End-of-Life Care

In this test section, the candidate is assessed on the ability to:

1. Evaluate a client's ability to cope with end-of-life interventions – An inability to cope can manifest as anger, anxiety, guilt and depression.

2. Identify the end-of-life needs in a client – End-of-life needs can be physical, psychosocial and spiritual. Physical needs include anorexia, dehydration and pain. Psychosocial needs include family support and belonging. Spiritual needs include prayer, meditation and other religious activities.

3. Provide psychosocial support to the family – Family support can come in the form of extended visits to the client, family and group therapy and teaching the client grief-coping mechanisms.

4. Educate the client's relatives and staff on end-of-life care – A nurse must educate the staff and client's relatives on the nursing care plan used to care for the client.

Kubler Ross Theory of Grief

The Kubler Ross theory of grief is also known as the Five Stages of Grief.

This theory is used to describe the sequence of emotions experienced by end-of-life clients and clients who have lost a loved one. They include denial, anger, bargaining, depression and acceptance. This theory was created by Elisabeth Kubler-Ross in 1969.

The five stages include:

1. Denial – In this stage, the client refuses to accept the diagnosis of a terminal illness. The client believes that the diagnosis is false.
2. Anger – In this stage, the client's denial gives way to anger. The client becomes frustrated and angry because the progression of the terminal illness forces him/her to realize that the diagnosis is real. The client may lash out at close individuals like caregivers and health workers.
3. Bargaining – In this stage, the client entertains the hope for a supernatural phenomenon. The client attempts to bargain for an extension of life in exchange for a lifestyle change. For example, the client might bargain to be happy, loving and kind, or fix a strained relationship in exchange for extended life.
4. Depression – In this stage, the client is depressed because the reality of mortality begins to dawn on him/her. In this stage, the client may refuse to talk, eat or have people around.

5. Acceptance – In this stage, the client accepts mortality as an inevitable end. In this stage, the client is calm, reflective and his/her emotions are stable.

Family Dynamics

In this section, the candidate is evaluated on the ability to:

1. Identify factors that affect family dynamics – Some of these factors include substance abuse, psychiatric disorders, religious and cultural views and socioeconomic status.

2. Assess parenting techniques – Parenting techniques in terms of discipline should be assessed by an RN to reduce the risk of abuse.

3. Encourage group and family therapy – Family therapy is important to help family members cope with stressors, which can include caring for a family member with a chronic and debilitating illness or who is terminally ill.

4. Identify teaching resources for assisting the family – The nurse should suggest teaching materials and resources that can help improve a family's dynamics.

5. Assist the client in integrating new members of the family – The nurse may teach blended families, adoptive parents and new mothers.

Grief and Loss

In this section, the candidate is evaluated on the ability to:

1. Assist the client in the grieving process – To do this, the RN must apply his/her knowledge of the different stages of grief. For example, Kubler Ross' Stages of Grief include shock and disbelief, denial, guilt, anger and bargaining, depression and loneliness, reconstruction and acceptance.

2. Assist the client in coping with loss – This involves the use of therapeutic communication techniques and provision of physiological and spiritual care.
3. Provide resource materials to help a client in the grieving process – These resources can make it easier for the client to reach acceptance.

Mental Health Concepts

In this section, the candidate is assessed on the ability to:

1. Identify the clinical features of impaired cognition – These features include but are not limited to memory loss, altered personality, depression and aggression.
2. Identify the clinical features of mental illness – Some of these features include but are not limited to sensory hallucinations, depression, mania, delusion and others.
3. Recognize the use of defense mechanisms – These defense mechanisms are used by the client to cope with stressful events.
4. Apply the principles of psychopathology to mental health care – These principles help an RN to prioritize and tailor a care plan to a client's needs. The needs should be prioritized according to urgency.
5. Evaluate the client for mood and personality changes, cognition, and reasoning – These changes are usual for clients with dementia and other forms of psychosis.
6. Evaluate a client's compliance with a treatment plan – Drug compliance, nurse-client interaction and mood are indicators used to evaluate a client's compliance with a treatment plan.

Religious and Spiritual Influences on Health

In this section, the candidate is assessed on the ability to:

1. Identify the religious and spiritual needs of the client – An RN can do this either by observation or by asking the client directly about his/her spiritual needs. For example, a nurse caring for a Muslim client should consider the position of the client's bed.

2. Assess the religious and spiritual factors affecting care – An RN is responsible for providing spiritual care to clients. Doing this requires an ability to identify the client's unique spiritual needs that affect care. For example, a client who is a Jehovah's Witness may object to treatment plans involving blood and blood transfusions.

3. Evaluate the interventions created to meet the client's needs – After providing care, a nurse should evaluate the success of these interventions in meeting the client's spiritual needs.

Sensory/Perceptual Alterations

In this section, the candidate is assessed on the ability to:

1. Identify the factors surrounding the appearance of the symptoms – This includes identifying the time, place and nature of the stimuli surrounding the symptoms. For example, auditory symptoms are more likely to occur in an environment that is filled with activity.

2. Assist clients in developing interventions for dealing with sensory hallucinations – These interventions include but are not limited to following safety protocols, creating an environment with minimal stimuli, educating

clients on procedures and treatment plans, frequently assessing clients and keeping clients' activities as routine as possible.

3. Provide nursing care for a client with hallucinations – Some nursing care includes the use of sedatives like benzodiazepines, therapeutic communication techniques and cognitive-behavioral therapy.

4. Provide reality-based diversions – This includes the use of techniques that attempt to orient the client to time, place and person.

Stress Management

In this section, the candidate is assessed on the ability to:

1. Identify potential stressors to a client – These stressors can be physical elements like light, noise, temperature change and overcrowding. These stressors can also be triggered by religious and cultural factors.

2. Recognize verbal and nonverbal signs of stressors – These include identifying signs and symptoms of stress, observing for abnormalities in laboratory investigations and observing a client's demeanor, body language and other nonverbal cues.

3. Create interventions to reduce stressors – These interventions can be pharmacological or non-pharmacological. For example, pharmacologic interventions include the use of drugs for therapeutic outcomes. Non-pharmacologic interventions include the provision of nursing care and the use of alternative therapies like meditation, deep breathing, acupuncture and others.

4. Educate clients on stress management techniques – As appropriate, clients should be educated on the benefits and proper use of stress management

techniques like deep breathing, massage, exercise, imagery, hypnosis and biofeedback.

Psychotherapy

Also known as talk therapy, psychotherapy is used to help clients cope with neurotic and psychotic illnesses. Psychotherapy can be used with medications or used alone to manage a variety of mental illnesses. Some types of psychotherapy include:

1. Cognitive Behavioral Therapy (CBT) – This form of psychotherapy helps clients identify harmful thought patterns and replace them with positive ones. CBT is used to manage a variety of mental disorders like depression, anxiety, stress disorders and eating disorders.

2. Interpersonal Therapy – This form of psychotherapy is a short form of treatment used to help clients identify underlying and worrisome issues. Some of these issues include grief, resentment and conflict in the family, workplace and relationships. It is also used to teach clients how to express their emotions better and communicate with others.

3. Dialectical Behavior Therapy – This form of psychotherapy is used to help clients regulate their emotions. It is used to manage clients with suicidal ideations, severe depression, eating disorders, borderline personality disorder and PTSD.

4. Psychodynamic Therapy – This form of psychotherapy is used to manage clients whose mental behavior is influenced by childhood experiences and who have inappropriate thoughts that are subconscious and repetitive. The therapist helps the client become more self-aware and change negative thought patterns to positive ones.

5. Psychoanalysis – This is an advanced form of psychodynamic therapy, usually done by a psychologist.
6. Supportive Therapy – This form of psychotherapy is used to give encouragement and support to clients who suffer from depression, low self-esteem, anxiety and other forms of neurosis. In this therapy, the client is encouraged to develop and use resources like coping mechanisms for improved social relationships.

Substance Use

In this section, the candidate is assessed on the ability to:

1. Assess a client with drug and alcohol dependency – An RN should assess a client's symptoms, history of drug or alcohol use and associated risk factors like genetics, mental disorder and family dynamics. The nurse should also assess the client for toxicity and withdrawal symptoms.
2. Provide care to clients with symptoms of withdrawal or toxicity – This includes the use of pharmacological interventions and the provision of nursing care to improve the client's nutrition, hydration and toileting.
3. Inform the client of the treatment plan and interventions – The client must be informed of the available interventions for managing addictions and withdrawal symptoms.
4. Encourage the client to participate in support groups – Support groups are a form of cognitive-based therapy. Examples of these groups include Alcoholics Anonymous and Narcotic Anonymous.

Substance Abuse Disorders

Substance abuse disorder is also known as drug-use disorder. It is the persistent use of drugs despite the harm and consequences. These drugs also include the use of alcohol.

The severity of substance abuse disorders varies from mild and moderate to severe.

Some of the terms used in addiction and dependence include:

1. Addiction – This is a biopsychosocial disorder in which the client compulsively seeks to achieve the desired effect despite harm.
2. Dependence – A state in which the client develops withdrawal symptoms when he/she ceases to use a substance.
3. Drug withdrawal – These are symptoms that occur when someone no longer utilizes the drug he/she was dependent on.
4. Physical dependence – These are somatic and physical symptoms that develop when a client stops taking a substance.
5. Psychological dependence – These are psychological and emotional withdrawal symptoms that develop when a client stops taking a drug.
6. Addictive drug – This is a drug that is both rewarding and reinforcing.
7. Addictive behavior – This is a behavior that is both rewarding and reinforcing.

Support Systems

In this section, the candidate is assessed on the ability to:

1. Assist the family in caring for a client with impaired cognition – This includes educating the client's family on the nature and progression of the disease and the medical interventions used to improve outcomes. The nurse should educate the client's family on the teaching and learning resources available to them.

2. Encourage the client to collaborate with the health team – This is necessary for providing client-centered care and reducing the risk of morbidity and mortality.

Therapeutic Communication

In this section, the candidate is assessed on the ability to:

1. Comprehend verbal and nonverbal communication – This includes assessing the client's ability to speak English proficiently, assessing the need for an interpreter and assessing the client's cognitive level in reference to age.

2. Use therapeutic communication techniques – There are many therapeutic techniques used to encourage clients to express themselves. Therapeutic communication techniques signify acceptance and respect for the client. As a nursing process, therapeutic communication is discussed in chapter 2.

3. Evaluate the effectiveness of communication techniques – Effective communication techniques make a client comfortable and relaxed. They also promote self-awareness and self-responsibility.

Therapeutic Environment

In this section, the candidate is assessed on the ability to:

1. Identify external factors that can impact a client's recovery – These factors include stressors which can be physical, physiological, social, religious and

economic. These factors include the nature of the client's family dynamics and support systems.

2. Provide therapeutic environments for clients – RNs should provide a therapeutic environment by eliminating all forms of physical and psychological hazards that interfere with a client's recovery.

Chapter 6: Physiological Integrity

This section includes four subsections: basic care and comfort, pharmacological and parenteral therapies, reduction of risk potential and physiological adaptation.

A. Basic Care and Comfort

This subsection makes up about 6-12% of the test. In this subsection, the candidate is evaluated on assistive devices, elimination, mobility and immobility, non-pharmacological comfort interventions, nutrition, oral hydration, personal hygiene, rest and sleep.

Assistive Devices

The candidate is assessed on the ability to:

1. Assess a client with functional impairments – The nurse should assess impairments in terms of walking, speech, vision and hearing. Further professional assessments should then be made by qualified health personnel. For example, an ophthalmologist should be consulted to assess a visual impairment.
2. Assess a client's ability to use assistive devices – Some of these assistive devices include walking devices like canes, walkers, wheelchairs and crutches. Auditory assistive devices include things like hearing aids.
3. Educate clients on the proper use of assistive devices – For example, a client should be educated on the importance of posture and alignment in using walking devices.

Elimination

The candidate is assessed on the ability to:

1. Evaluate and manage the client with a change in elimination – Clients with constipation, diarrhea and urinary and fecal incontinence should be evaluated to rule out causes and risk factors. After that, they must be managed according to the diagnosis. For example, clients with constipation should be given stool softeners and osmotic laxatives to improve bowel motility. They should also be prescribed a high-fiber diet.

2. Irrigate the bladder, eyes and ears – Bladder irrigation should be done in cases of hematuria, pyuria and necroturia. Ear irrigation should be done for ear infections, while eye irrigation is necessary for conjunctivitis caused by microbes or irritants.

3. Provide skin care to incontinent clients – An incontinent client is at risk for dermatitis caused by continuous exposure to water and salts from the urine and feces. Some skin-care measures include the use of petroleum jelly and other skin sealants, along with keeping the affected area dry at all times.

4. Use alternative methods to encourage elimination – A client with urinary incontinence may benefit from a urethral catheter.

5. Evaluate management outcome – This includes an assessment of both objective and subjective data. For example, a client who has a urethral catheter for a bladder outlet obstruction should be evaluated in terms of the amount of urine voided into the urinary bag and also for complications like hematuria, post-catheterization diuresis, urinary tract infections and pain.

Enemas

An enema is the process of administering a liquid into the rectum so as to administer drugs or stimulate bowel motility.

Types of Enemas

1. Cleansing Enemas – In this process, a water-based solution is used to stimulate the movement of the colon. Normal saline is used for a cleansing enema because its isotonic properties reduce the client's risk for an electrolyte imbalance. There are three types of cleansing enemas: large-volume enemas, small-volume enemas and disposable enemas.

A. Large-Volume Enemas – A large-volume enema is done to relieve the client's colon, and also to prep the colon for a diagnostic procedure. About 500-1000 mls of normal saline is used. The bag of saline is raised to about 18 inches above the anus.

B. Small-Volume Enemas – This enema is used to cleanse the lower part of the colon, the sigmoid colon. About 500 mls of normal saline is used, and the bag is raised no more than 12 inches above the anus.

2. Prepackaged Disposable Enemas – This is the most common enema used in hospitals. A common brand is the Fleet enema. This enema is used to relieve constipation and also to prep the client for diagnostic procedures. Unlike the other enemas listed above, this enema is hypertonic and contains gut stimulants like Bisacodyl and sodium phosphate. The hypertonic solution draws fluid into the bowel and softens the impacted feces. These enemas are available in 150 ml and 37 ml sizes.

3. Oil Retention Enemas – This enema is used to soften impacted feces. The enema comes in sizes of about 90-120 mls. Clients should be encouraged to retain the enema solution for about an hour. This enema is used in conjunction with a cleaning enema.

4. Return Flow Enemas – Also known as a Harris Flush, this enema is used to remove intestinal gas and stimulate peristalsis. A large volume of water is administered in increments of 100-200 mls. The fluid is then drawn by lowering the enema container below the level of the anus. This brings out the flatus along with the fluid.

5. Cooling Enemas – This is not a common procedure. This enema is done to rapidly cool the temperature of clients with hyperpyrexia. The temperature must be assessed before, during and after the procedure.

6. Rectal Administration of Drugs – Enemas can also be used to give rectal drugs. These drugs soothe the gut mucosa, correct electrolyte imbalance or treat infections.

Complications of Enemas

1. Perforation – To reduce the risk of perforation, enemas are contraindicated in clients with intestinal obstruction, paralytic ileus and radiotherapy.

2. Fluid Imbalance – Hypertonic solutions can cause dehydration when there is a massive movement of fluid from the intravascular space to the bowel. The hydration status of a client should be assessed before commencing an enema.

3. Electrolyte Imbalance – Hyponatremia is a complication of large-volume enemas. Large amounts of water can move into the intravascular space and cause dilutional hyponatremia. Also, Fleet enemas increase the risk of hyperphosphatemia, especially in the elderly.

4. Infection – To reduce the risk of infection, sterilized equipment must be used for an enema.

5. Rectal Prolapse – This is a complication of chronic enemas.

Mobility and Immobility

The candidate is evaluated on the ability to:

1. Identify the different complications of immobility – Most complications of immobility are chronic. Some of these include pressure sores, muscle atrophy, bone demineralization, stress-induced gastric ulcers, orthostatic pneumonia, constipation, urinary tract infections and urolithiasis.

2. Assess clients' mobility, gait, strength and motor skills – The range of motion of a client's limbs is assessed when the client stands up, changes from a sitting position to standing and walks.
3. Provide measures to maintain skin integrity and prevent skin breakdown – These include measures to prevent pressure sores, some of which include two-hourly turning of the client, eliminating shearing and friction, keeping the body dry and physiotherapy.
4. Apply the principles of nursing procedures and psychomotor skills when caring for immobile clients – These principles are physiological concepts applied to prevent further complications in immobile clients. For example, measures like adequate water intake and the use of prophylactic urinary antiseptics can reduce the risk of urinary tract infection.
5. Apply and remove orthopedic devices – Examples of these devices include splints, braces, casts and traction devices.
6. Apply devices used to increase venous return – These devices work by increasing venous pressure. Examples of these devices include compression stockings and automatic sequential compression devices.
7. Maintain the client's traction device – Traction devices are used to maintain the alignment of fractured bones. Examples include Hamilton Russell Traction and Buck's Skin Traction.
8. Institute measures to improve circulation – These measures include positioning and repositioning of the client, routine exercises, mobilization and physiotherapy.
9. Evaluate the client's response to these interventions – Factors used to measure the improvement of an immobile client include increased range of

joint motion and flexibility, improvement of pressure sores, increased ambulation and increased muscle mass.

Non-Pharmacological Comfort Interventions

The candidate is evaluated on the ability to:

1. Evaluate the client's need for alternative and complementary therapy – Some of these alternative therapies include meditation, prayer, acupuncture, magnets, chiropractic services, Reiki and music therapy.
2. Assess the client's need for palliative measures – End-of-life clients and clients with chronic diseases and complications need palliative measures. Palliative measures aren't curative. They are therapeutic measures used to make clients comfortable. Examples include pain management, food and nutrition, counseling and grief management for family members.
3. Assess the client's need for pain management – Pain is both objective and subjective. Pain can come in many forms. For example, pain can be superficial, deep, somatic, psychological, acute, chronic, diffused, localized and so on.
4. Recognize differences in perception to pain – Perception of pain varies from client to client. Factors that influence perception of pain include ethnicity, religious beliefs, cultural values, age, sex, cognitive function and family support.
5. Apply the principles of pathophysiology to non-pharmacological palliative measures – For example, an end-of-life client may be anorexic, incontinent, depressed, agitated and restless.
6. Counsel and respect the client's choice of palliative measures – Apart from counseling a client on existing palliative measures, an RN should be open to

the client's choice of palliative care. For example, a client may request alternative therapies like prayer and pastoral care.

7. Assess the client's response to non-pharmacological measures – Non-pharmacological measures of pain management include acupuncture, aromatherapy, meditation, yoga and body massage. Clients may demonstrate better outcomes after using these therapies.
8. Assess the outcome of palliative care measures – Some of these outcomes include improved demeanor and mood, improved appetite and increased ambulation.

Nutrition and Oral Hydration

The candidate is assessed on the ability to:

1. Evaluate the client's ability to eat – These include assessing the client's appetite, mechanical factors preventing food intake, personal food choices, religious practices, lifestyle choices and therapeutic interventions.
2. Assess the client for food and drug interaction – These drug interactions can be synergistic or antagonistic. For example, clients on warfarin therapy are counseled to avoid foods rich in vitamin K, because vitamin K is an antagonist of warfarin.
3. Recognize the client's food choices – Food choices are dependent on the client's cultural values, religious beliefs and socioeconomic status, among others. For example, a Jewish client may refuse to eat non-kosher foods.
4. Assess the client's hydration status – This includes an assessment of objective data like blood pressure, skin turgor, capillary refill, pulse rate, urine output and water intake. Severe dehydration puts a client at risk for hypovolemic shock.

5. Assess the client's nutritional and calorie intake – This includes measuring objective data like weight, body mass index, assessing signs of deficiencies in hair, nails, skin and oral activity, and measuring calorie intake.
6. Encourage the client's independence in eating – A nurse should encourage a client to select meal plans. The nurse should also teach the client to use assistive devices like weighted plates, food guards, tip-proof drinking glasses and scoop dishes.
7. Provide nutritional supplements as required – Some of these nutritional supplements include iron therapy for iron deficiency anemia, calcium supplementation for bed-ridden clients, high-protein diets for clients with protein-losing enteropathy, restricted salt intake for clients with kidney disease, etc.
8. Give intermittent tube feedings when indicated – Intermittent tube feedings are indicated for clients with a gastrointestinal disorder, swallowing disorder, severe anorexia, burns or unconsciousness. They are also indicated for clients undergoing chemotherapy or radiotherapy.
9. Assess the impact of disease on a client's nutritional status – Acute and chronic illnesses have a significant impact on a client's nutritional status. For example, most inflammatory states are characterized by increased catabolism of protein, glycogen, fats, vitamins and minerals. In cancer, there is an activation of tumor necrosis factors and other cell mediators that stimulate catabolism.

Personal Hygiene

The candidate is assessed on the ability to:

1. Evaluate a client's personal hygiene habits – This includes evaluation of bathing, oral care, nail care, foot care and perineal care. Factors that influence personal hygiene include religious beliefs, ethnicity, socioeconomic status, cognitive and physiological function and age, among others.
2. Educate clients on personal hygiene practices – Clients should be educated on the importance of good personal hygiene in preventing diseases of the skin, respiratory and gastrointestinal systems. For example, personal hygiene reduces the incidence of fungal and parasitic infections of the skin.
3. Perform postmortem care – An RN should also perform postmortem care such as the removal of all indwelling devices like nasogastric feeding tubes, urethral catheters and intravenous lines. An RN is responsible for washing the deceased client's body and covering it with a cloth.

Rest and Sleep

The candidate is evaluated on the ability to:

1. Assess a client's need for rest – A nurse should know the estimated amount of sleep required in each age group. For example,

A. 0-2 years require about 12-17 hours of sleep.

B. 3-5 years require 11-14 hours of sleep.

C. 6-12 years require 9-11 hours of sleep.

D. 13-17 years require about 8-10 hours of sleep.

E. Young adults and middle-aged adults require 7-9 hours of sleep.

F. Older adults over 65 years require 7-8 hours of sleep per night.

2. Apply the principles of pathophysiology to rest and sleep interventions – An RN should provide interventions for factors that prevent the client from sleeping. For example, it can be difficult for a client to sleep if he/she is in pain. The nursing intervention here is to provide analgesia. A client with obstructive sleep apnea can find it difficult to sleep and may need a CPAP machine.

3. Schedule the client's activities to encourage adequate rest – For example, a nurse can schedule family visits in the morning when a client is alert and active. This can give the client more time to rest in the evening and at night.

B. Pharmacological and Parenteral Therapies

This subsection makes up about 12-18% of the overall test. The topics covered include adverse effects, contraindications, side effects and interactions of drugs, blood and blood products, central venous access devices, dosage calculations, expected actions and outcomes, medication administration, parenteral and intravenous therapies, pharmacological pain management and total parenteral nutrition.

Adverse Effects, Contraindications, Side Effects and Interactions of Drugs

The candidate is evaluated on the ability to:

1. Identify contraindications to a medication – This includes contraindications for pregnant women, lactating mothers, hypertensives, those with kidney and liver disease and others.

2. Identify drug-drug interactions of prescribed medications – Drug-drug interactions can delay or increase the metabolism of drugs. For example,

drug-drug interactions can occur between drugs that are metabolized by cytochrome P450 enzymes.

3. Identify symptoms of an allergic drug reaction – Symptoms can include rashes, hypotension, nausea, vomiting, diarrhea and others. At the onset of these reactions, the implicated drug should be stopped immediately.
4. Evaluate the client for side effects and adverse effects of medications – Unlike adverse effects, side effects are unexpected for both the clinician and the client. Typically, side effects are not dose-related, while adverse effects are. Observing and assessing physiological data is important in diagnosing adverse and side effects.
5. Educate the client on common side effects and adverse effects of prescribed medications – The client should be educated on all potential side effects and adverse effects of a drug before beginning to take the medication.
6. Inform the primary health-care provider of side effects and contraindications of medications and parenteral therapy – The primary health-care provider should be educated on the side effects, adverse effects, contraindications and potential drug-drug interactions of the prescribed drugs.
7. Monitor the client for anticipated interactions – As soon as the prescription is started, vital signs should be monitored for possible drug interactions.
8. Document the client's response to actions taken to counteract side effects and adverse effects of medication – In the event of adverse and/or side effects, interventional therapy should be started. Clients' responses to interventions should be recorded.

Blood and Blood Products

The candidate is assessed on the ability to:

1. Identify the client prior to a blood transfusion – This includes confirmation of the client's blood group, serology results and blood products to be transfused. This confirmation should be done by at least two nurses, using the two-person verification technique.

2. Identify the appropriate venous access for blood transfusion – Wide-bore cannulae, i.e., size 16 or size 18, are used for transfusion of blood and blood products. Doing so reduces the risk of hemolysis.

3. Document the necessary information on the administration of blood products – Documentation is important for both medical and legal reasons.

4. Evaluate the client's response to blood transfusion – The client should be assessed for potential transfusion reactions. Clinical features of transfusion reaction include hives, fever, chills, rigor and hypotension.

Blood Products

Whole blood is not routinely used in medical practice; instead, blood products are used. Blood products are therapeutic components prepared from human blood. They include:

1. Red Blood Cells – Red blood cells are used to treat hemorrhages and inefficient oxygen perfusion into tissues. Indications for a red blood cell transfusion include symptomatic anemia, hemorrhagic shock and acute sickle cell crisis.

2. Plasma – Fresh frozen plasma is used to reverse the hemorrhagic effects of anticoagulants.

3. Platelets – Platelet transfusion is used to prevent hemorrhages in clients with thrombocytopenia. Cryoprecipitate is used to treat hypofibrinogenemia, which often occurs in massive hemorrhage and consumptive coagulopathy.

Complications of Blood Transfusions

Blood transfusion complications can be acute or delayed.

1. Acute Complications of Blood Transfusion – Acute complications occur within 24 hours of a blood transfusion. They include acute hemolytic reaction, anaphylactic reaction, coagulopathies caused by massive transfusion, febrile non-hemolytic reaction, transfusion-associated circulatory overload, urticarial reaction, transfusion-related acute lung injury and sepsis.

2. Delayed Complications of Blood Transfusion – These transfusion reactions occur at least 24 hours after the blood transfusion. They can take days, months or years. Examples are delayed hemolytic reaction, post-transfusion purpura, iron overload, microchimerism, over-transfusion and transfusion-related immunomodulation.

Central Venous Access Devices

The candidate is assessed on the ability to:

1. Educate the client on the indications of venous access – A client should be educated on the indications of venous access. Some of these indications include fluid resuscitation and administration of intravenous antibiotics.

2. Educate clients on the importance of care of venous devices – Intravenous access puts a client at risk of sepsis. Precautions taken to reduce the incidence of sepsis include daily cleaning of the ports with an antiseptic solution, changing peripheral lines no less than 48 hours after their insertion and the use of gloves when administering intravenous drugs and fluids.

3. Set up venous access devices – An RN should set up peripheral venous accesses using a suitable size of canulae. Wide-bore cannulae are used for acute resuscitation and blood transfusion, while narrow-bore cannulae are

used for already stable patients, and also for giving intravenous maintenance fluids.

4. Care for a client with a central venous access device – Care includes daily cleaning of ports with antiseptic solutions, use of face masks and sterile gloves when accessing a central line, flushing the lines before and after use, changing dressings every 48 hours and replacing the injection cap on each lumen every week. Care should also be taken to prevent an air embolism.

Dosage Calculations

The candidate is assessed on the ability to:

1. Calculate doses of medications – This skill involves the knowledge and application of measurement systems used in pharmacology. Measurements include the use of teaspoons, tablespoons, cups, pints, drops, gallons and pounds. The apothecary measurement has weight measurements like pounds, drams, ounces and grains. The metric measurement is the most popular measuring system used in pharmacology. It includes cubic milliliters, cubic centimeters, kilograms, milligrams and micrograms.
2. Use clinical decision-making when calculating doses – RNs should apply their knowledge of the principles of clinical pharmacology and pathophysiology when administering drugs. This reduces the risk of errors.

Expected Actions and Outcomes

The candidate is assessed on the ability to:

3. Gather information on a client's prescription – This involves consulting reliable sources like the *Physician's Desk Reference*, a formulary, a drug handbook, a pharmacist or a reliable internet source.

4. Use clinical decision-making to evaluate expected effects and outcomes – An RN should monitor a client for expected therapeutic responses. This involves collation and assessment of physiological data like temperature, respiration, blood pressure, hematologic reports, radiology reports and so on. To do so, the RN applies the principles of pathophysiology, pharmacology and pathology.
5. Evaluate the long term effects of medications – This involves monitoring a client's adherence and compliance to drugs, monitoring side and adverse effects, therapeutic response to prescribed medications and the cumulative effects of medications.

Medication Administration

The candidate is assessed on the ability to:

1. Educate a client on medications – This involves educating the client on all the necessary pharmacokinetics and pharmacodynamics properties of a drug.
2. Educate a client on self-administration of medications – This is necessary for outpatient administration of drugs either at home or at home centers. For example, an RN should educate a diabetic client on how to self-administer insulin, and an asthmatic client should be taught how to use a metered-dose inhaler.
3. Prepare and administer medications – An RN should know how to prepare intravenous, intramuscular and other forms of medications. To do so, the nurse must be knowledgeable about the principles of the ten rights of medication: medication, dose, time or frequency, patient, route, client education, documentation, right to refuse, assessment and evaluation.

4. Review important data before administering medications – A nurse should review a medication order before administering a drug. Information in the medication order includes the client's name, the date and time of the order, the name of the drug, the dose of the drug, the route of administration, the frequency of the dose and the signature of the ordering physician.
5. Mix medications when necessary – An RN should know that only compatible drugs can be mixed. For example, a diabetic client can safely mix NPH insulin and regular insulin in one syringe.
6. Administer and document medications given by common routes – Common routes of administration include oral, sublingual, topical, transdermal, ophthalmic, intravenous, vaginal and rectal.
7. Administer and record medication given by parenteral routes – Documentation is necessary for medical and legal reasons.
8. Conduct medication reconciliation – This process is done to reduce the incidence of medication errors. In this process, all the client's drugs, including prescription drugs, over-the-counter drugs, herbal remedies, nutritional and dietary supplements, vaccines and radioactive drugs are compiled under a list of current medications and newly prescribed medications. The two lists are then evaluated for inconsistencies. The client is then educated on the list of newly prescribed drugs.
9. Titrate the dosage of medications based on assessment and ordered parameters – Drug dosages are adjusted depending on therapeutic responses and the physician's order. For example, some antihypertensives are adjusted according to a client's blood pressure.
10. Dispose of unused medications – Unused medications must be disposed of according to a hospital's policy. If a controlled substance is discarded, there

should be a second witness. Also, the name of the discarded drug must be recorded.

11. Evaluate the client's medication orders – Medication orders must be assessed by an RN. Some components that are evaluated include the accuracy of the order, known allergies, vital signs data and important laboratory findings.

Parenteral and Intravenous Therapies

The candidate is assessed on the ability to:

1. Identify veins for various therapies – RNs must identify and select veins for various intravenous therapies. For example, veins on the upper extremities are preferred to veins on the lower extremities. Veins on a client's non-dominant arm are preferred to veins on the dominant arm. Areas distal to a thrombosed or infiltrated site should be avoided. The side of a client's mastectomy, paralysis and dialysis should also be avoided.

2. Educate the client on the importance of intermittent parenteral fluid therapy – Clients must be updated on the importance of various parenteral therapies. Also, they should be taught to inform the nurse when they experience pain or notice swelling of the insertion site.

3. Apply the principles of nursing when administering parenteral therapy – This involves the application of mathematics, psychomotor skills and nursing procedures.

4. Prepare a client for the insertion of an intravenous catheter – A client should be informed of the purpose of the catheter, the procedure for inserting the catheter, the care of the insertion site and when to notify the nurse of complications.

5. Monitor an infusion pump – This involves monitoring a pump's flow rate. This is done by calculating the flow rate with the infusion rate of the pump device.

6. Assess a client's response to intermittent parenteral fluid therapy – A client's physiological data must be observed to assess therapeutic outcomes. It also involves assessing the client for possible complications like infiltration, extravasation, phlebitis, hematoma, embolus formation and fluid overload.

Pharmacological Pain Management

The candidate is assessed on the ability to:

1. Assess a client's need for administration of a PRN pain medication – PRN drugs are given when the nurse notes pain in a client. Pain can be assessed using the PQRST method, using a pain scale or assessing the behavioral and physiological features of pain, i.e., tachycardia, diaphoresis and hypertension.

2. Administer and document pain medications – Pharmacological pain medications are given in consideration of certain factors like age, weight, diagnosis and underlying medical conditions that can affect the metabolism and excretion of these drugs.

3. Administer controlled drugs within specific guidelines – The administration of narcotics requires that legal requirements be met, such as the signature of the nurse picking up the drug, securing narcotics in a locked place and a two-witness evaluation of wasted and discarded narcotics.

4. Evaluate the client's response to pain medications – This involves an assessment of both objective and subjective data. Objective assessment of pain includes observation of physiological data like heart rate and blood pressure. Subjective assessment of pain includes the use of the pain scale.

Total Parenteral Nutrition

The candidate is evaluated on the ability to:

1. Identify side effects of TPNs – Some of these side effects include pneumothorax, hydrothorax, hemothorax, infection, fluid overload, hyperglycemia and embolism.
2. Educate the client on the indications of TPN – Like all medical interventions, the client must be informed of the indications of TPN. TPN is usually used for clients with a negative nitrogen balance as seen in clients with cancer, AIDS and severe burns.
3. Use the principles of pathophysiology in administering TPN – This involves assessing the client's need for TPN. This involves assessment of the client's body weight, serum glucose, protein and electrolytes and other vital signs.
4. Administering and evaluating the client's response to TPN – An RN must be aware of the conditions for administering TPN. For example, TPN feedings must be refrigerated before they are given. TPN administration is an aseptic procedure that requires thorough adherence to asepsis. Precautions must be taken to prevent air embolisms. For example, a nurse should encourage a client to perform a Valsalva maneuver to prevent an air embolism. Also, the TPN tubing must be changed every 24 hours.

C. Reduction of Risk Potential

This subsection makes up about 9-15% of the overall test. In this subsection, the candidate is assessed on changes and abnormalities in vital signs, diagnostic tests, laboratory values, the potential for alteration in body systems, potential for complication from surgical procedures and health alteration, the potential for complications of diagnostic tests, treatments and procedures, system-specific assessments and therapeutic procedures.

Changes and Abnormalities in Vital Signs

In this section, the candidate is evaluated on the ability to:

1. Evaluate and respond to changes in vital signs – Vital signs are objective physiological data obtained from a client. They include respiratory rate, heart rate, blood pressure, temperature, urine output and oxygen saturation. Vital signs are used to assess the baseline function of a client's system. They are also used for the early detection of pathophysiology.

2. Apply the principles needed to perform nursing procedures – Critical thinking and clinical judgment are necessary for obtaining vital signs from patients. For example, temperature is measured either as axillary, oral, aural or rectal. Blood pressure is measured on the arm. Respiratory rate is measured by observing the rise and fall of the anterior chest wall and monitoring the activities of the subcostal and intercostal muscles.

3. Apply the principles of pathophysiology in measuring vital signs – An RN should be proficient in the principles of pathophysiology in order to interpret data from vital signs measurement. For example, respiratory rates vary according to age group:

A. Neonates: 30-60 cycles per minute.

B. Infants: 20-40 cycles per minute.

C. Toddlers: 20-30 cycles per minute.

D. School-Aged Children: 16-24 cycles per minute.

E. Adolescents and Adults: 12-20 cycles per minute.

4. Evaluate invasive monitoring data – Invasive monitoring data includes intracranial pressure, pulmonary artery pressure and other types of hemodynamic data. These data require proficiency in the application of the principles of pathophysiology and psychomotor skills.

Diagnostic Tests

In this section, the candidate is assessed on the ability to:

1. Apply the principles of nursing procedures and psychomotor skills when caring for clients undergoing diagnostic testing – Diagnostic tests can be invasive or non-invasive. Regardless of the nature of the test, an RN is responsible for performing general tasks like:

A. Confirming the doctor's order for the diagnostic tests.

B. Confirming the client's identity.

C. Procuring informed consent from the client after educating him/her on the indications and possible complications of the procedure.

D. Adhering to universal guidelines.

E. Accurately labeling specimens.

F. Properly preserving and transporting specimens.

2. Compare the client's diagnostic findings with pre-test results – An RN must compare the results of procedures with the pre-test results and report any abnormalities to the ordering physician.

3. Perform fetal heart monitoring – This involves the use of a Pinard horn, a sonicaid or a cardiotocograph to monitor the fetal heart. Fetal bradycardia and tachycardia are early signs of fetal distress.

4. Monitor results of maternal and fetal diagnostic results – This involves procedures like a non-stress test, amniocentesis and ultrasound. These procedures are done to diagnose congenital abnormalities which may or may not be compatible with life.

5. Evaluate the results of diagnostic tests and intervene as needed – After a procedure is performed, the results must be compared with normal physiological values. Abnormalities should then be reported to the ordering physician.

Laboratory Values

In this section, the candidate is examined on the ability to:

1. Identify laboratory values of various blood investigations – This includes evaluating the results of hematologic investigations, serum electrolytes, urea, creatinine, acid blood gas and other metabolic profiles like glucose, protein, lipids, cholesterol and so on.

2. Compare the client's laboratory values with normal laboratory values – An RN should be able to compare the client's results with normal laboratory values and intervene as needed.

3. Educate the client on the importance of laboratory tests – Like all medical treatments, informed consent must be obtained after educating the client on the benefits and potential complications of a procedure.

4. Obtain specimens for diagnostic testing – This includes obtaining blood from intravenous access, and obtaining other specimens like urine, sputum, throat swabs, vaginal swabs and wound swabs from clients. Some of these are aseptic procedures that have strict guidelines on collection.

5. Monitor the client's laboratory values – Some clients need serial monitoring of their laboratory values. For example, a diabetic client will need serial monitoring of fasting and random blood sugar. A client with a kidney injury will need serial monitoring of potassium, sodium, bicarbonate, urea and creatinine.

6. Notify primary health-care providers of laboratory test values – The primary health-care provider should be updated and informed of the result of the monitoring.

Potential for Alteration in Body Systems

In this section, the candidate is assessed on the ability to:

1. Identify clients at risk for aspiration – Clients who are at risk of aspiration include clients with decreased levels of consciousness, nasogastric tubes, impaired lower esophageal sphincters, endotracheal tubes, impaired cough or gag reflexes and dysphagia.

2. Identify clients at risk of skin breakdown – Factors that promote skin breakdown include immobility, malnutrition, fecal and urinary incontinence, impaired tissue perfusion, exposure to mechanical forces like friction and shearing, exposure to moisture, radiation, hypothermia and hyperthermia.

3. Identify clients at risk for insufficient vascular perfusion – Risk factors for impaired vascular perfusion include diabetes, hypovolemic shock, anemia, immobility, decreased cardiac output and hypoxia, among others.

4. Educate the client on prevention methods for disease complications – Secondary prevention methods are used to reduce the risk of complications and disabilities. These prevention methods are specific to certain diseases. For example, the risk of a diabetic foot ulcer in a diabetic client is reduced

when the client is educated on foot-care principles like wearing the right size of shoes, not walking around with bare feet, preventing foot moisture, inspecting the feet daily and controlling serum glucose.

5. Compare the client's current clinical data to baseline clinical data – This is done to evaluate the client's response to medical management.
6. Monitor the client's output for baseline changes – The client's output data can include the output of urine, vomitus, stools and drainage from a pleural effusion, fistulae, hemothorax or surgical drain. This data is used to evaluate pathophysiological processes.

Potential for Complication from Surgical Procedures and Health Alteration

In this section, the candidate is assessed on the ability to:

1. Apply the principles of pathophysiology in monitoring complications – Complications can arise from numerous physiologic processes like inflammation, hemolysis, metabolic derangement, degeneration and so on.
2. Assess the client's response to postoperative interventions in preventing complications – This includes interventions for complications like wound dehiscence, aspiration, sepsis, paralytic ileus, immobility and impaired venous return, among others.

Potential for Complications of Diagnostic Tests, Treatments and Procedures

In this section, the candidate is assessed on the ability to:

1. Assess a client for an abnormal response following a diagnostic test – Some diagnostic tests have side effects and complications. For example, cardiac

catheterization can cause dysrhythmia. Chemotherapeutic drugs can cause alopecia, dermatitis, stomatitis and immunosuppression.

2. Apply the principles of nursing when caring for a client with a risk of complications – Examples of these principles include monitoring the pulse rate of a client with a cast to detect compartment syndrome, proper positioning of a client with a tracheostomy to prevent aspiration and two-hourly turning of a bedridden client to prevent pressure ulcers.
3. Monitor a client at risk of bleeding – This includes but is not limited to monitoring a client on anticoagulant therapy, monitoring a post-op client, monitoring a client with leukemia, esophageal varices, stress ulcers and others.
4. Position the client to prevent complications following treatment and procedures – For example, a client should be positioned in a supine position after a spinal tap. A client with pulmonary edema should be placed in the cardiac position to relieve lung congestion.
5. Insert a nasogastric tube – An RN is responsible for inserting a nasogastric tube for clients with clear indications for it.
6. Insert a urethral catheter – Urethral catheterization is a sterile procedure done to help clients void urine.
7. Maintain tube patency – An RN must maintain the patency of a variety of tubes like nasogastric tubes, chest tubes and urethral catheters.
8. Provide care for a client undergoing electroconvulsive therapy – Examples of care provided include maintaining the client on NPO at least six hours prior to a procedure to reduce risk of aspiration, securing intravenous access for

administration of emergency intravenous drugs and monitoring clients for seizure, among others.

9. Evaluate responses to procedures and treatments – This involves collation and assessment of both subjective and objective data, before and after treatment.

System-Specific Assessments

In this section, the candidate is assessed on the ability to:

1. Examine the client for abnormal peripheral pulses after a procedure – An indication of these includes a cast application, peripheral artery disease, diabetes mellitus and crush injury, among others.
2. Examine the client for abnormal neurological status – This involves assessment of the Glasgow Coma Scale, cranial nerve function, muscle tone, power and reflexes.
3. Examine the client for peripheral edema – Peripheral edema occurs when there is an accumulation of fluid in the extracellular space. Edema occurs when there is a reduction in the oncotic pressure as seen in kidney disease like nephrotic syndrome. It can also occur when there is an increased hydrostatic pressure, as seen in right-sided heart failure.
4. Examine the client for hypoglycemia/hyperglycemia – Clients with diabetes mellitus are at risk of both hypoglycemia and hyperglycemia. Other causes of hypoglycemia include sepsis, malnutrition, use of insulin and antidiabetic agents. Causes of hyperglycemia include Cushing syndrome, excess growth hormone secretion, prolonged steroid use and others.

5. Identify the factors that delay wound healing – These factors include protein deficiency, diabetes mellitus, obesity, peripheral artery disease, dehydration and zinc deficiency, among others.

6. Evaluate changes in the client's outcome – As always, nurses are expected to assess the therapeutic outcome of their clients.

7. Perform focused assessment – This involves performing a detailed systemic examination for a diagnosis. For example, clients at risk for kidney injury should have an assessment of the urogenital system.

Therapeutic Procedures

In this section, the candidate is assessed on the ability to:

1. Evaluate the client's response to recovery from anesthesia – This involves assessing the client's recovery from local, regional and general anesthesia. Vital signs such as blood pressure, oxygen saturation, pulse rate, respiratory rate and cardiac rhythm are continuously monitored.

2. Educate a client about treatment and procedures – The client should be educated on a treatment before informed consent is sought. Important components such as the indication of the treatment, benefits of the treatment, complications of the treatment and alternative therapies available should all be communicated to a client.

3. Educate the client on home-care management – Clients who are discharged from acute facilities to care homes should be educated on home care principles like care of tracheostomies, colostomies, surgical wounds, ulcers and others.

4. Apply cautionary guidelines to avoid injury when moving a client with a musculoskeletal injury – This involves the use of guidelines and principles

that prevent further worsening of musculoskeletal injuries. For example, log-rolling is used for clients with a fracture of the spine.

5. Monitor the client before, during and after a procedure – This involves collation and assessment of both subjective and objective data, pre-, intra- and postoperatively.

6. Monitor the functioning of therapeutic devices – Therapeutic devices include chest tubes, nasogastric tubes, surgical drains, bladder irrigation systems, etc. An RN must assess these devices for leaks, kinks, disconnections and obstructions.

7. Provide preoperative, intraoperative and postoperative care – Preoperative care includes a comprehensive physical assessment and clinical history, retrieving results of laboratory investigations, administering preoperative medications, obtaining informed consent, etc.

8. Provide intraoperative care – This includes positioning the client correctly for the surgery/procedure, preparing a sterile field, counting sponges, sharps and other surgical instruments and assessing the client's vital signs.

9. Provide postoperative care – This includes monitoring the client's vital signs, assessing and managing pain and monitoring all therapeutic devices.

10. Provide preoperative and postoperative education – The client must be educated on the principles of care provided pre-, intra- and postoperatively. The aim of education is to keep the client informed, allay fears and encourage active participation in care management.

D. Physiological Adaptation

Physiological adaptation includes alterations in body systems, fluid and electrolyte imbalances, hemodynamics, illness management, medical emergencies, pathophysiology and unexpected responses to therapies.

Alterations in Body Systems

The candidate is assessed on the ability to:

1. Evaluate a client's adaptation to disease – This involves assessing a client's approach to coping mechanisms, crisis intervention, support systems, family dynamics, grief and loss and end-of-life care.

2. Assess tube drainage during illness – This includes assessing wound drainage, respiratory drainage, chest tube drainage, etc. Data such as quantity, color, consistency and other characteristics of the drainage must be recorded.

3. Assess the client for clinical features of adverse effects to radiotherapy – This involves assessing the client for common side effects like alopecia, dental caries, fatigue, immunosuppression, strictures, bone marrow suppression, cataracts, dermatitis and so on.

4. Identify potential prenatal complications – This includes assessing women for complications like cardiac disease, sexually transmitted infections (STIs), hypertension, anemia, diabetes mellitus, current drug history and exposure to radiation.

5. Identify the clinical features of infectious diseases – This includes assessing clients for signs and symptoms of infectious diseases. Cardinal signs include fever, chills, rigor, cough, and fast breathing for respiratory infections, and vomiting, diarrhea, bloody stool, abdominal pain and weakness.

6. Apply the principles of pathophysiology and nursing psychomotor skills in caring for a client – For example, when caring for a diabetic, an RN should apply psychomotor skills and the principles of pathophysiology in controlling a client's blood sugar and educating the client on the proper use of a glucometer, how to self-administer insulin and how to avoid complications.

7. Educate the client on disease management – This includes educating the client on all secondary and tertiary prevention methods to treat disease and avoid complications.

8. Assist with invasive procedures – An RN must assist doctors and other health-care professionals with invasive procedures like spinal taps, catheterization of a central line, needle biopsies, intubations, thoracenteses and chest tube insertions.

9. Implement and monitor phototherapy – Phototherapy is used to treat psoriasis and neonatal unconjugated hyperbilirubinemia. The nurse must monitor the use of phototherapy machines to reduce the risk of complications like hypothermia, conjunctivitis and bronze baby syndrome.

10. Treatment for adverse effects of radiotherapy – The adverse effects of radiotherapy are managed symptomatically. For example, a female client with alopecia should be given psychological support and counseled to try alternate hairstyles like wigs or short hair. To prevent further hair loss, the client should be counseled to wash her hair with a mild shampoo and advised to protect her hair from sunlight.

11. Maintain the optimal temperature of the client – The nurse should evaluate a client for risk of hypothermia and hyperthermia. For example, risk factors for hyperthermia include infections, hyperthyroidism, use of psychotropic drugs

and exposure to hot temperatures. The risks for hypothermia include hypothyroidism, trauma, diabetes and exposure to very cold environments.

12. Monitor and care for a client on a ventilator – This includes monitoring for complications like aspiration, nosocomial pneumonia, fluid retention, hyperventilation, hypoventilation, oxygen toxicity and so on. To prevent these complications, the nurse should take measures such as continually monitoring the client's vital signs and making prompt nursing interventions when necessary.

13. Assess wounds for infection – This involves assessing clients for symptoms like redness, heat, fever, fatigue, nausea and vomiting, abdominal cramping and diarrhea, discharge from the wound site and others. Nurses should assess clients for these signs and make prompt interventions to reduce morbidity.

14. Manage a client on peritoneal dialysis – A nurse should provide care pre-, intra- and post-dialysis. Pre-dialysis care includes an assessment of a client's physiological data like weight, blood glucose, urea, creatinine and hematocrit. During dialysis, a nurse monitors a client's input and output. After dialysis, the nurse evaluates the client's weight, blood pressure, glucose and other laboratory values.

15. Perform suctioning – Suctioning is indicated for clients with excessive secretions in the airway. Suctioning can be done in the oral, nasopharyngeal, endotracheal and tracheal cavities. Before suctioning, a nurse should take precautionary measures such as identifying and obtaining informed consent from the client, pre-oxygenating the client, using sterile gloves and maintaining strict asepsis, using adequate lubrication and, if possible, analgesia.

16. Provide ostomy care – RNs care for clients with bowel and tracheal ostomies. The nursing care plans for such clients include education on home care, risk factors for complications, clinical features of complications and interventions to reduce mortality.

17. Care for a client with infectious disease – This includes initiating the infection protocol depending on the source of the infection, providing therapeutic relief and commencing antimicrobial therapy.

18. Provide pulmonary hygiene – These are interventions done to reduce secretions in the respiratory airway. For example, a client with a tracheostomy should be encouraged to cough to clear the airway. Other interventions like suctioning and providing warm, humidified air can also be done.

19. Provide care for a client in labor – This includes monitoring both maternal and fetal vital signs, providing nursing care to reduce pain and discomfort and making prompt nursing interventions when the need arises.

20. Provide care for the client with raised intracranial pressure – A client with raised intracranial pressure is at risk of brain herniation and death. To reduce this risk, precautionary principles must be followed. Some of these include raising the head of the bed to about 30 degrees to improve venous drainage and using intravenous mannitol to reduce cerebral edema.

21. Provide post-op care – This task requires a sound grasp of pathophysiology, nurse psychomotor skills and a knowledge of the numerous nursing care plans and nursing interventions available to clients recovering from a variety of surgeries.

22. Remove sutures and staples – An RN is also responsible for removing sutures and staples post-op. Before doing so, the wound must be assessed for

dehiscence and infection. The nurse should then follow precautionary guidelines like cleansing the wound with a topical antiseptic, clipping the sutures with a pair of sterile scissors and swabbing the skin with antiseptic after the sutures are removed.

23. Evaluate the client's response to radiotherapy – This involves evaluating the client for therapeutic responses and possible side effects post-radiation.

24. Assess a client's response to surgery – Part of the postoperative care provided by a nurse involves assessment and evaluation of a client's physiological data.

25. Assess a client's response to treatment of an infectious disease – A client's physiological data like temperature and respiratory rate must be assessed before, during and after the start of antimicrobial therapy.

Fluid and Electrolyte Imbalance

The candidate is assessed on the ability to:

1. Identify the clinical symptoms of a client with fluid and electrolyte imbalance – This involves assessing a client for signs of edema, mild, moderate and severe dehydration, and various electrolyte imbalances like hyper and hyponatremia, hyper and hypokalemia, hyper and hypocalcemia and so on.

2. Apply the principles of pathophysiology in caring for a client with fluid and electrolyte imbalance – A nurse must apply knowledge of etiology, risk factors, clinical features and complications in caring for a client with a fluid and electrolyte imbalance.

3. Evaluate a client's response to fluid and electrolyte correction – A nurse should evaluate a client's response to therapeutic intervention by collecting and interpreting physiological data like level of consciousness, cardiac rhythm, blood pressure and laboratory data.

Water and Electrolyte Imbalance

Sixty percent of the body's weight is made up of water. Two-thirds of this amount is stored in the intracellular space, while the remaining third is found in the extracellular space, which comprises the intravascular space and interstitial space.

The daily fluid requirement is calculated using the metric system. It includes 100 ml of fluid for the first 10 kg, 50 ml of fluid for the second 10 kg and 10 ml of fluid for each additional kilogram of body weight.

1. Dehydration – A client is dehydrated when he/she loses a significant amount of his/her body's water volume required for homeostasis. Dehydration can be mild, moderate or severe. Causes of dehydration include fever, prolonged sun exposure, hyperglycemia, burns and gastroenteritis. Clinical features of dehydration include lethargy, headache, muscle weakness, dry mouth, dry skin, sunken eyes, low blood pressure, increased heart rate and unconsciousness.

2. Hypokalemia – This is used to describe a potassium level that is below 3.5 mmol/L. Causes of hypokalemia are gastroenteritis, diseases of the adrenal glands, laxatives, total parenteral nutrition, diuretics and stimulants. Symptoms of hypokalemia include paralytic ileus, constipation, weakness, fatigue, muscle cramps, muscle twitching and arrhythmia.

3. Hyperkalemia – This is a term used to describe a serum potassium level that is above 5.5 mmol/L. Causes of hyperkalemia include the use of potassium-sparing diuretics, chronic kidney disease, rhabdomyolysis and hypoaldosteronism. Clinical features of hyperkalemia include numbness, muscle weakness, tingling sensation, fatigue and cardiac arrest.

4. Hyponatremia – This is used to describe a serum sodium that is less than 135 mmol/L. Causes of hyponatremia include congestive heart failure, SIADH,

drinking too much water, Addison's disease, dehydration and use of stimulants like amphetamines, diuretics and antidepressants. Clinical features of hyponatremia include nausea, vomiting, headaches, confusion, fatigue, restlessness, seizures and coma.

5. Hypernatremia – This is used to describe serum sodium levels that are above 145 mmol/L. Causes include dehydration, diabetes insipidus, Conn's Syndrome, excess salt intake, ingestion of hypertonic fluids like seawater and excess consumption of soy sauce. Clinical features of hypernatremia include thirst, seizures and coma.

Hemodynamics

The candidate is assessed on the ability to:

1. Assess the client for decreased cardiac output – Decreased cardiac output is a precursor for shock. When a client's cardiac output is decreased, it means that the client's heart is unable to meet the oxygen demands of tissues. In shock, there is decreased oxygen perfusion into the tissues, leading to a cascade of metabolic derangement and subsequent death. Features of shock include hypotension; tachypnea; cold, clammy extremities; altered consciousness and reduced urinary output.

2. Identify cardiac rhythm abnormalities – A nurse should have the skill to interpret ECG readings. This involves determining the heart rate, determining the cardiac rhythm, assessing the P wave, assessing the PR interval, assessing the QRS complex and making a diagnosis.

3. Apply principles of pathophysiology to interventions in treating cardiac abnormalities – An RN should be able to apply knowledge such as the

physiology and pathophysiology of cardiac output, blood pressure, ejection fraction, resistance to blood flow and others.

4. Educate the client on strategies to manage decreased cardiac function – This involves symptomatic management of features of reduced cardiac output as listed above. It also involves rapid intervention on cardiac diseases to improve the client's quality of life and reduce mortality.
5. Monitor and maintain arterial lines – A nurse should be able to maintain arterial lines by reducing the risk of infection, embolism and hemorrhage.
6. Manage a client with a pacemaker – Clients on continuous cardiac monitoring should be either monitored by nurses or a telemetry technician. However, regardless of whoever does the monitoring, a nurse is responsible for interpreting the results of the ECG and providing interventions when necessary.
7. Manage a client on hemodialysis – This includes the provision of pre-, intra- and post-dialysis care as listed above.
8. Manage a client with altered hemodynamics – A nurse is responsible for providing prompt interventions for clients with clinical features of shock and impaired tissue perfusion.

Illness Management

The candidate is assessed on the ability to:

1. Apply the principles of pathophysiology to disease management – A nurse must be proficient in the required knowledge of pathophysiology needed to make a clinical judgment and perform the necessary nursing interventions.

2. Report abnormal data immediately – A nurse is responsible for interpreting laboratory results, identifying abnormal data and immediately reporting it to the ordering physician.
3. Educate the client on his/her disease condition – An RN must also educate the client on the primary, secondary and tertiary levels of preventing the disease, its progression and subsequent disabilities and complications.
4. Perform gastric lavage – Gastric lavage is indicated as an intervention for emergencies such as drug poisoning, gastrointestinal bleeding and drug overdoses. An RN must be equipped with the psychomotor skills and knowledge of human anatomy to carry out this task.
5. Provide continuity of care – An RN must initiate, maintain and monitor a client from the point of first contact, all the way to discharge.
6. Manage a client with impaired ventilation – To do this, a nurse must assess a client with impaired ventilation by assessing physiological data like respiratory rate and oxygen saturation. Interventions should then be carried out to improve clinical data.
7. Evaluate the treatment plan of a client with a medical diagnosis –An RN must evaluate the nursing care plan of the client and make the necessary adjustments to achieve the desired therapeutic outcome.

Medical Emergencies

The candidate is assessed on the ability to:

1. Apply the principles of pathophysiology in caring for a client with an emergency – An RN must follow the principles of airway, breathing and circulation to stabilize clients in acute and emergency states.

2. Apply principles of nursing procedures and psychomotor skills in caring for a client with an emergency – Nursing procedures that are useful for a client in an emergency state include CPR, defibrillation, intubation and gastric lavage, among others.
3. Explain emergency interventions to a client – If a client is unstable, informed consent can be obtained from the caregiver, family member or significant other. If these aren't applicable, implied consent should be obtained.
4. Perform emergency care procedures – A nurse must be skilled at performing nursing procedures that can save the client in an acute state.
5. Provide care for wound disruption – A wound can eviscerate or dehisce depending on certain factors. These two conditions are surgical emergencies that require prompt intervention to reduce the risk of hemorrhage and infections.
6. Evaluate and document therapeutic outcomes to interventions – After initiating an emergency intervention for a client, the client's response must be assessed by evaluating the vital signs, laboratory results and other data.
7. Pathophysiology – the candidate is assessed on the ability to:

   Identify pathophysiologic processes related to an acute or chronic condition – This ability requires an understanding of etiology, risk factors, clinical signs and symptoms, complications, diagnostic findings and treatment of both acute and chronic diseases.

   Understand the general principles of pathophysiology – An RN is expected to have an understanding of the principles of the stages of infection, the signs and symptoms of infection, the phases of bacterial growth, the phases of infection and all the concepts of immunity.

Unexpected Responses to Therapies

The candidate is assessed on the ability to:

1. Assess the client for adverse response to interventions – These include adverse effects to surgical, pharmacologic and non-pharmacologic interventions. Some of these adverse effects include iatrogenic trauma and lacerations; tube leakage, dislodgement, and consequent pneumothorax and hemothorax; iatrogenic infections, as seen in urinary tract infections and pneumonia; needle-prick injuries and other forms of biohazards.

2. Recognize the clinical features of adverse complications and intervene promptly – An RN must quickly identify the signs and symptoms of infection and hemorrhage related to these adverse effects and make prompt interventions.

3. Encourage the recovery of a client with an adverse response to therapy – A nurse must identify and eliminate the factors that can interfere with a client's recovery. For example, in caring for a client with an iatrogenic urinary tract infection caused by prolonged catheter use, the nurse must reassess the client's need for a urethral catheter and may decide to choose another method to help the client void urine.

Test 1

1. All of the following are sources of information for a scholarly journal except ...

A. Research reports

B. Primary sources

C. Secondary sources

D. Personal beliefs

2. All of the following are examples of qualitative research except ...

A. Field research

B. Grounded theory research

C. Experimental research

D. Case study research

3. A study is conducted to compare the sensitivities of the most popular glucometers used in home-care centers. Which of the following is the independent variable in the study?

A. Sensitivities of glucometers

B. Brand of glucometer

C. Hospice centers

D. None of the above

4. Which of the following is the dependent variable in the home-care center study?

A. Sensitivities of glucometers

B. Brand of glucometers

C. Hospice center

D. None of the above

5. Which of the following factors greatly influences the pharmacodynamics of drugs in the elderly?

A. Compliance

B. Hepatic drug clearance

C. Alcohol consumption

D. Oxygen saturation

6. All of the following are unfavorable outcomes of polypharmacy except ...

A. Drug-drug interaction

B. Adverse effects

C. Non-compliance

D. Narrow therapeutic index

7. You are auscultating a client's precordium with a stethoscope. Which of the following is correct?

A. High-pitched sounds are assessed with the bell

B. Low-pitched sounds are assessed with the diaphragm

C. A diastolic murmur is a low-frequency sound

D. An apex beat is a low-frequency sound

8. Which of the following hematological tests is not necessary prior to a red blood cell transfusion?

A. Hematocrit

B. Clotting profile

C. Serology

D. Blood grouping and cross-matching

9. Which of the following principles of x-rays is false?

A. Radiopaque tissues are white on the film

B. Radiolucent tissues are dark on the film

C. Air is a radiopaque substance

D. Radiopaque tissues absorb more x-rays than radiolucent tissues

10. Which of these best describes collaborative nursing interventions?

A. They are interdependent nursing interventions implemented with other health-care professionals

B. They are nursing interventions done under the supervision and directive of a medical doctor

C. They are nursing interventions implemented by a team of two to four nurses

D. They are nursing interventions implemented by the leader of a nursing team

11. Which of these is correct concerning hospital-acquired pneumonia?

A. Symptoms occur more than 72 hours after admission in patients with no evidence of infection prior to admission

B. It is also known as nosocomial pneumonia

C. Fungal infections are a common cause

D. Prophylactic use of systemic steroids is indicated

12. Which of these best describes the primary nursing care model?

A. Nurses are paired and attached to individual clients

B. Nurses are assigned duties and report individually to a single nurse

C. Nurses move from unit to unit

D. A single nurse is the primary caregiver of the client

13. In modular nursing care, the nursing staff is allocated based on which of the following components?

A. The client's ethnicity

B. The client's geographic location

C. The client's disease category

D. The client's age

14. Which of the following ethnicities is most at risk of developing post-surgical keloids?

A. Hispanic American

B. Native American

C. African American

D. Jewish American

15. Which of the following ethnicities is most likely to avoid direct eye contact during a nurse-patient interaction?

A. Chinese American

B. Native American

C. African American

D. Jewish American

16. The following conversation ensues between a nurse and a client who is being managed for nicotine addiction.

Client: My father died of lung cancer because he smoked a lot of cigarettes. I should stop smoking, but it's so hard.

Nurse: You are worried that your addiction will give you lung cancer.

What communication technique is this?

A. Offering self

B. Probing

C. Paraphrasing

D. Giving recognition

17. The following conversation ensues between an elderly client in a home center and a nurse.

Client: My children should be here to see me by now. I know they are busy at work, but they promised to show up early this time.

Nurse: I notice you've stopped knitting your sweater.

What communication technique is this?

A. Restating

B. Recognition

C. Making observation

D. Paraphrasing

18. Which of the following ethical principles is correct?

A. Justice is synonymous with beneficence

B. Nonmaleficence means doing no intentional harm to clients

C. Fidelity is synonymous with faithfulness

D. Accountability means the nurses are accountable to the doctors

19. Nurses are obliged to follow ethical guidelines provided by all the following regulatory bodies except which of these?

A. American Nurses Association

B. American Medical Association

C. The World Medical Association

D. The World Nurses Association

20. Which of the following is a primary disease prevention method?

A. Routine handwashing

B. Intravenous antibiotics for pyelonephritis

C. Chest physiotherapy for a sickle cell client

D. Blood transfusion for a hemophiliac

21. You are to assess the bowel sounds of a client on his second day post-operation for appendicitis. Which of the following is false?

A. A hypoactive bowel makes one bowel sound in three to five minutes

B. Hypoactive bowel sounds can indicate an intestinal obstruction

C. Borborygmi are a form of hyperactive bowel sounds

D. Bowel sounds are heard to the right of the umbilicus

22. Your client is two days post-operation for a herniorrhaphy. Which of these conditions puts him at risk for delayed wound healing?

A. Cobalamin deficiency

B. Diabetes mellitus

C. A BMI of 21 kg/m^2

D. Serum sodium of 138 mmol/L

23. You are a nurse working in a hospital with a BFHI. The hospital implements all the following steps to encourage successful breastfeeding except ...

A. Give infants no food or drink other than breast milk unless indicated

B. Encourage breastfeeding on demand

C. Help mothers initiate breastfeeding within 24 hours of birth

D. Give no pacifiers or artificial nipples

24. A new mother is struggling to position her infant for breastfeeding. When repositioning her, you will use all of the following guidelines for proper positioning and attachment except ...

A. Position the baby's whole body to face the mother's chest

B. The baby's head should rest on the mother's elbow or arm

C. The baby's nose should be opposite the mother's areola

D. The baby's ears, shoulders and hips should be in a straight line

25. The colostrum is rich in which of these antibodies?

A. IgA

B. IgG

C. IgM

D. IgE

26. A client with a common cold should be advised to adhere to all of the following cough guidelines except ...

A. Cover the mouth and nose with a tissue when coughing

B. Cough or sneeze into the upper sleeve if a tissue isn't available

C. Cough into the hands and wash them off immediately if a tissue isn't available

D. Dispose of single-use tissues immediately

27. Which of these meal plans is suitable for a client with gluten intolerance?

A. Mixed-grain cereal with milk and blueberries

B. Tofu and mixed vegetable salad with quinoa

C. Spaghetti with shrimp sauce and orange juice

D. Avocado and cheese bagel sandwiches

28. You are caring for a hospice patient who will probably pass away in the next 48 hours. What theory of grief is suitable for this client's relatives?

A. Warden's theory of grief

B. Lewin's theory of grief

C. Engel's theory of grief

D. Kubler Ross' theory of grief

29. Which of the following is true about a child with attention deficit hyperactivity disorder?

A. The child prefers routines and inanimate objects

B. The child will benefit from a structured and controlled environment

C. The child has a mental IQ of 20

D. The child has a history of stealing and lying

30. You are caring for a group of teenage girls with bulimia nervosa and anorexia nervosa. Which of these psychotherapy interventions is most suitable?

A. Behavioral therapy

B. Aversive conditioning

C. Flooding and implosion

D. Supportive therapy

31. Your client is a five-year-old female who was brought into the emergency room by her parents. They complain that she has begun wetting herself recently. You learn that this behavior started after the birth of her baby brother. What defense mechanism is this?

A. Reaction formation

B. Regression

C. Sublimation

D. Repression

32. Which of these defense mechanisms is commonly seen in paranoid disorders?

A. Regression

B. Projection

C. Repression

D. Reaction formation

33. A clinic has a philosophy of focusing on and strengthening the existing abilities of its clients rather than focusing on the progression of diseases. This clinic is modeled after which of these models of disability?

A. The biomedical model

B. The social model

C. The cognitive model

D. The pathological model

34. A twelve-week gravid client is expected to experience all of the following physiological changes except ...

A. Mood swings

B. Constipation

C. Pica

D. Frequent urination

35. Your client is a cancer patient who used to be on prescription Oxycontin. He no longer has a need for prescription drugs. However, he presented to the emergency unit with symptoms of Oxycontin overdose. Your client is suffering from which of these disorders?

A. Substance abuse

B. Physical dependence

C. Addiction

D. Psychological dependence

36. A bedridden client will benefit from which of these?

A. An orthopedic bed

B. An air bed

C. A cardiac bed

D. A recumbent bed

37. An incontinent patient will benefit from which of the following?

A. A urethral catheter

B. Diapers

C. A bedpan

D. A cystostomy

38. To reduce calcium loss in a bedridden client, which of the following interventions is necessary?

A. Increase fluid intake

B. Turn the client every two hours

C. Engage the client in weight-bearing exercises

D. Commence muscle physiotherapy

39. Which assistive device is useful to a high school teacher with aphasia?

A. A bell

B. A hearing aid

C. A pad and a pen

D. A pointer

40. Assistive dressing tools for a client with Parkinson's disease include all of the following except ...

A. Zipper pulls

B. Button hooks

C. Elastic shoelaces

D. Slippers

41. You are about to insert a nasogastric tube into the nostrils of a client with left hemispheric CVD. All of the following principles are beneficial except ...

A. Lubricate the tip of the tube with a water-based lubricant

B. Place the patient in a High Fowler's position

C. Anesthetize the back of the client's throat with aerosol anesthesia

D. Place the patient in the Sims position

42. A client with myocardial infarction caused by atherosclerosis will benefit from which of the following meal plans?

A. Foods rich in plant fiber

B. Highly starchy foods

C. Foods rich in protein

D. Foods high in unsaturated fat

43. How many hours should neonates sleep?

A. 14–17 hours

B. 10–11 hours

C. 8–9 hours

D. 6–7 hours

44. You are to administer 50 mg of medication. If 20 mg is in 1 ml, how many milliliters will you administer?

A. 2 ml

B. 2.5 ml

C. 1.5 ml

D. 3 ml

45. You are to give 250 mg of an oral tablet. If 100 mg is in one tablet, how many tablets will you give?

A. 2.5 tablets

B. 2 tablets

C. 3.5 tablets

D. 3 tablets

46. Which of these is not a likely complication of TPN?

A. Embolism

B. Hyperglycemia

C. Diarrhea

D. Sepsis

47. The O negative blood group is also known as?

A. Universal red blood cell donor

B. Universal plasma cell donor

C. Universal whole blood donor

D. Universal platelet donor

48. A patient with Type B negative blood is to receive Type O negative blood. Which of these is true?

A. The recipient has B antigens, D antigens and A antibodies

B. The donor has D antigens but no A and B antigens

C. The recipient has C antigens, Y antigens and A antibodies

D. The donor has only A and B antibodies

49. When administering IM medications, all of the following are landmarks for identifying the administration site on the gluteal muscle except ...

A. The lesser trochanter

B. The greater trochanter

C. The anterior superior iliac spine

D. The iliac crest

50. All of the following drugs have a narrow therapeutic window except ...

A. Lithium

B. Digoxin

C. Penicillin

D. Acetaminophen

51. A client scheduled for an examination under anesthesia for suspected cervical malignancy will need all of the following blood results reviewed by the anesthetist except ...

A. Serum bicarbonate

B. Hematocrit

C. ESR

D. Serum potassium

52. Which of the following parameters is not useful for a client on warfarin therapy?

A. INR

B. PT

C. PTT

D. PCV

53. Which of the following cannulae is appropriate for a neonate?

A. Size 18G

B. Size 16G

C. Size 20G

D. Size 26G

54. Concerning the A blood group type, which of the following is true?

A. It has A antigens and A antibodies

B. It is compatible with an AB blood donor

C. It is compatible with an AB recipient

D. It has A antigens in its plasma

55. Which of the following intravenous fluids is not used for emergency resuscitation?

A. Dextran

B. Hartmann's solution

C. Normal saline

D. Dextrose water

56. Which of the following is true concerning the extravasation of drugs?

A. It is typical of IM medications

B. It is associated with vesicant drugs

C. It is associated with non-vesicant drugs

D. A treatment modality is the application of a warm compress

57. Which of these is true about phlebitis?

A. It is usually associated with alkaline solutions

B. It can be managed by the application of a hot compress

C. It is commonly caused by solutions with low osmolarity

D. Chemotherapy drugs are a likely cause

58. Concerning infiltration, which of the following is correct?

A. 50% dextrose water is a likely cause

B. 0.9% normal saline is a likely cause

C. IV paclitaxel is a likely cause

D. IV vancomycin is a likely cause

59. A client with liver cirrhosis complains of constipation. Nursing interventions should be performed to avoid which of the following complications?

A. Intestinal obstruction

B. Hepatic encephalopathy

C. Rectal bleeding

D. Gastroenteritis

60. A 24-year-old primigravida at 22 weeks presents for her routine prenatal care with a blood pressure of 140/90 mmHg. The woman's urinalysis shows two pluses of protein in her urine. Which of the following statements is correct?

A. She is at risk of developing preeclampsia

B. She is at risk of developing eclamptic fits

C. She is at risk of going into cardiogenic shock

D. The fetus is at risk of a congenital anomaly

61. A client with ESRD develops a sudden onset of fast breathing. His pulse is about 90 beats in a minute. Blood pressure is 130/80 mmHg. Partial oxygen saturation is 75%. What should your first response be?

A. Resuscitate the client with intravenous fluids

B. Resuscitate the client with a vasoconstrictor

C. Provide supplemental oxygen

D. Start cardiac massage

62. On presenting to the emergency unit, a client is noted to have an RBS of 24 mmol/L. His dipstick urinalysis revealed three pluses of glucose and three pluses of ketones. What should your first response be?

A. Give the client SC insulin

B. Hydrate the client with normal saline

C. Collect a urine sample for microscopy

D. Assess the client's level of consciousness

63. A six-month-old male presents to the neurology clinic for follow-up. Which of the following guidelines is correct pertaining to OFC measurements?

A. Macrocephaly is an OFC that is greater than or equal to the 95th percentile

B. Macrocephaly is an OFC that is greater than or equal to the 99th percentile

C. The landmarks for measuring this client's OFC are the glabella and the occiput

D. Microcephaly is an OFC that is less than the fifth percentile

64. A nine-year-old male client presents to the endocrinology clinic for follow-up. Which of these guidelines is correct pertaining to BMI?

A. Obesity is a weight that is greater than or equal to the 95th percentile

B. Underweight is a BMI that is below the third percentile

C. BMI is measured in kilograms per square centimeter

D. BMI is a direct measurement of body fat

65. A client who is preparing to receive the next cycle of chemotherapy presents with a hematological report as follows:

PCV – 20%

Platelets count – 150,000 mcL

Total WBC – 6,000 mcL

Which of these actions is appropriate?

A. Commence chemotherapy

B. Give prophylactic antibiotics before commencing chemotherapy

C. Transfuse with fresh frozen plasma

D. Transfuse with red blood cells

66. A client with CKD presents to the clinic with this electrolyte report:

Potassium – 6.0 mmol/L

Sodium – 135 mmol/L

Creatinine – 600 mmol/L

Urea – 35 umol/L

This client will benefit from which of the following treatments?

A. A dextrose insulin infusion to treat hyperkalemia

B. Hemodialysis

C. An intravenous diuretic

D. A potassium-sparing antihypertensive

67. Which of these blood reports is abnormal and should be reported to the doctor?

A. Potassium 3.6 mEq/L

B. Calcium 3.5 mEq/L

C. Sodium 135 mEq/L

D. Bicarbonates 25 mEq/L

68. Which of the following blood reports is abnormal and should be reported to the doctor?

A. Triglycerides 1.6 mmol/L

B. Cholesterol 6.5 mmol/L

C. HDL 28 umol/L

D. LDL 2.5 mmol/L

69. An orthopedic client with a scotch cast complains of numbness in his bandaged arm. Which of these is the most likely diagnosis?

A. Compartment syndrome

B. Orthopedic neuropathy

C. Phantom limb syndrome

D. Compression syndrome

70. Which of these clients has the greatest risk of developing pressure ulcers?

A. A diabetic client with an FBS of 6 mmol/L

B. A client with a GCS of 3

C. A client with left hemispheric ischemic CVD

D. A client with stage 2 Parkinson's disease

71. Hypocalcemia is least likely in which of the following clinical presentations?

A. An 80-year-old male with end-stage renal disease

B. A 5-year-old female with vitamin D insufficiency

C. A 34-year-old female with a total thyroidectomy

D. A 40-year-old female with a goiter

72. Which of the following is not a management option for a client with sickle cell anemia?

A. Hydroxyurea

B. Analgesia

C. Iron therapy

D. Chest physiotherapy

73. Cyanosis is least likely in which of the following clinical scenarios?

A. Carbon dioxide poisoning

B. Anemia

C. Tetralogy of Fallot

D. Polycythemia

74. Which of these isn't an example of active immunity?

A. A client with a history of chicken pox in early childhood

B. A client who has received a shot of homologous human globulin

C. A client who received a BCG vaccine in childhood

D. A six-week-old child who just received an IPV

75. Concerning type 2 diabetes mellitus, which of the following is correct?

A. It's a disease of adulthood

B. It's a disease of childhood

C. There is decreased insulin sensitivity

D. Insulin is the treatment of choice

76. A client with Cushing syndrome is least likely to have which of these?

A. Hyperglycemia

B. Hypertension

C. Hyperpigmentation

D. Obesity

77. In type 1 diabetes mellitus, clients are most likely to present to the endocrinology clinic with which of the following symptoms?

A. Polyphagia

B. Diabetic ketoacidosis

C. Polydipsia

D. Enuresis

78. A client has just had a total thyroidectomy for hyperthyroidism. He will benefit from which of the following supplements?

A. Magnesium

B. Calcium

C. Ascorbic acid

D. Cobalamin

79. A diabetic client complains of a pins-and-needles sensation in his feet. Which of the following foot-care tips is correct?

A. Use a foot antiperspirant daily

B. Moisturize soles, the dorsal surface and in between the toes daily

C. Soak feet in hot water for quick relief

D. Shave corns with a pumice stone or file

80. Which of these best explains why diabetic ketoacidosis is an endocrinology emergency?

A. Severe dehydration can cause hypovolemic shock

B. Excess blood glucose can trigger hemolysis

C. Excess blood sugar is a precursor to diabetic neuropathy

D. Excess blood sugar impairs the vascular supply to the kidneys

81. A client with a fasting blood sugar of 5.7 mmol/L has which of these conditions?

A. Impaired glucose tolerance

B. Diabetes mellitus

C. Hypoglycemia

D. Normal fasting glucose

82. A client with Parkinson's disease finds it difficult to button his shirt because he lacks which of the following neurotransmitters?

A. Serotonin

B. Dopamine

C. Acetylcholine

D. Epinephrine

83. A client presents to the emergency room with a severe head injury caused by a road traffic accident. On examination, he is discovered to have unequal eye pupils. What is this clinical sign called?

A. Miosis

B. Mydriasis

C. Anisocoria

D. Ptosis

84. Concerning miosis, which of the following is incorrect?

A. It can be a sign of opioid overdose

B. It is a parasympathetic response

C. It is a constriction of the pupils

D. It is part of the fight or flight response

85. A client presents to the emergency room with a history of severe headaches following a fall in the bathroom. The client is distressed because he can't remember how he got to the emergency room. However, he can remember the events before the fall. This client has which of the following conditions?

A. Anterograde amnesia

B. Retrograde amnesia

C. Mental block

D. Personality disorder

86. Concerning Horner's syndrome, which of the following is correct?

A. It's caused by a block to the parasympathetic pathway

B. It's caused by a block to the sympathetic pathway

C. Mitosis is a clinical sign

D. Excessive sweating is a sign

87. Which of the following is not a symptom of chronic liver disease?

A. Ascites

B. Jaundice

C. Cyanosis

D. Finger clubbing

88. Contact isolation is ideal for which of the following clients?

A. A pediatric client with measles

B. A female client with genital warts

C. A pediatric client with rotavirus infection

D. An adult client with pulmonary tuberculosis

89. All of the following clients are eligible for respiratory isolation except ...

A. A client with RSV

B. A client with measles

C. A client with aspiration pneumonitis

D. A client with meningococcal meningitis

90. A client with severe aplastic anemia is placed in reverse isolation. Which of the following is correct concerning reverse isolation?

A. It is a form of contact isolation for the immunosuppressed

B. It is a form of airborne isolation for the immunosuppressed

C. It is a form of isolation that protects a client from the environment

D. It is a form of isolation that protects the environment from the client

91. You are providing nursing care to a client with suspected pulmonary tuberculosis. What should your first safety measure be?

A. Wear eye goggles

B. Wash your hands

C. Wear a nose mask

D. Wear a protective gown

92. You are assessing the environment of an elderly patient to eliminate risks of a fall. Which of the following is not helpful?

A. Installing handrails

B. Installing proper lighting

C. Placing throw rugs in hallways

D. Installing grab rails

93. As a nurse, you are giving a health talk on sexually transmitted infections to a group of college students aged 18–25 years. Which of the following is true concerning STIs?

A. They can be prevented through hormone contraceptives

B. Examples include chlamydia, herpes and varicella zoster

C. They can be transferred through kissing

D. Bacterial vaginosis is a common example among females

94. A two-week-old neonate is receiving phototherapy for unconjugated hyperbilirubinemia. Which of the following complications is incorrectly matched to its preventive measure?

A. Retinal damage – eye cover

B. Overheating – monitor temperature

C. Dehydration – give adequate fluids

D. Bronze baby syndrome – keep phototherapy lights no more than 30.5 cm away from the neonate

95. Your client is scheduled to receive systemic radiation therapy for cervical cancer. Which of the following guidelines is incorrect?

A. Pregnant women are excluded from visiting this client

B. Children younger than 18 years are excluded from visiting this client

C. Visitors are to stay at least six feet away from the client's bed

D. Visitors are to stay no more than 30 minutes per visit

96. Your client is to receive ECT for severe depression. Which of the following complications is incorrectly matched to its preventive measure?

A. Bites and injuries – remove dentures

B. Aspiration – overnight fasting for at least six hours

C. Fractures – use a restraining vest

D. Confusion – give anxiolytics

97. Which of the following guidelines is correct in the prevention of hospital-acquired MRSA?

A. Use of droplet isolation measures

B. Use of prophylactic steroids for postoperative care

C. Immunization of all bedridden and chronic patients

D. Reduce the length of hospital admission

98. Which of the following is the most effective method in reducing the incidence of infectious diseases among schoolchildren?

A. Handwashing

B. Immunization

C. Social distancing

D. Health education

99. You are counseling the parents of a 10-month-old client with gastroenteritis. Which of the following is incorrect?

A. Handwashing reduces the risk of infection

B. Breastfeeding confers immunity to children

C. Rotavirus vaccine is a primary prevention method

D. Probiotics can prevent future occurrences

100. All of the following are stages of Kubler Ross' theory of grief except ...

A. Denial

B. Anger

C. Despair

D. Bargaining

Test 2

1. Concerning waste management and disposal, the yellow waste container is for disposing of which of the following drugs?

A. Cytotoxic drugs

B. Used syringes, catheters and urine bags

C. Used sharps

D. Human tissues

2. When disposing of biomedical waste, used sharps and needles should be disposed of in which of these containers?

A. Yellow

B. Red

C. Black

D. White

3. Which of the following methods is not useful in reducing hospital-acquired urinary tract infections?

A. Encourage patients to wash their hands before using the toilet

B. Limit the use of urinary catheters

C. Encourage patients to use bedpans

D. Increase the intake of fluids

4. Concerning the use of face masks, which of the following is incorrect?

A. Face masks protect from infectious aerosols and droplet nuclei

B. Face masks are used for contact isolation measures

C. Face masks should be worn over the nose and mouth

D. Single-use face masks should be disposed of when damp

5. All of the following are true about rooms with negative pressure except ...

A. Isolation rooms are examples

B. Air flows out of the room but not into it

C. Pressure in the room is lower than that of its surroundings

D. These rooms are used for a client with SARS

6. All of the following are true about rooms with positive pressure except ...

A. Pressure in the room is greater than that of the surroundings

B. These rooms are used for clients with immunosuppression

C. Air doesn't flow into the room

D. Autopsy rooms have positive pressure

7. You have just been handed a term neonate with mild meconium stain. The child is pink, with blue extremities. He has active, spontaneous movements and cries as you dry him with a towel. On auscultation, his heart rate is 120 bpm.

What is this child's Apgar score?

A. 7

B. 8

C. 9

D. 10

8. Based on the neonate's Apgar score, which of the following nursing interventions is appropriate?

A. Suction the nostrils with a suction bulb

B. Commence chest compressions

C. Commence CPAP

D. Give IV epinephrine

9. A pediatric client presents to the children's emergency room with acute Tylenol poisoning. All of the following guidelines are true except ...

A. Use activated charcoal if ingestion was less than four hours ago

B. Aspirate gastric contents through a nasogastric tube

C. Administer Mucomyst if ingestion was within eight hours

D. Disulfiram is the antidote of choice

10. All of the following are chronic complications of meningitis except ...

A. Epilepsy

B. Deafness

C. DIC

D. Hydrocephalus

11. You are an assistant preparing to receive a term male neonate delivered via Caesarean section. Which of the following is correct?

A. An Apgar score is given in the first and tenth minute of life

B. A pulse rate of 95 bpm has a score of 2

C. If the baby has pink skin and blue extremities, he is given a score of 1 for appearance

D. If the child grimaces, he has a grimace score of 2

12. All of the following are methods of stimulating this child's respiration except ...

A. Drying

B. Rubbing his back

C. Suctioning his mouth and nose

D. Giving a surfactant

13. A 19-year-old female client has just had a termination of pregnancy. All of the following are necessary medical interventions except ...

A. Providing contraception

B. HIV and STI screening and treatment

C. Vaccinating with Gardasil 9

D. Obtaining parental consent for contraception

14. A two-month-old pediatric patient presents as lethargic to the children's emergency room. The mother gives a history of prolonged vomiting and diarrhea. You make a diagnosis of severe dehydration secondary to gastroenteritis. This child has lost what percentage of his body's water volume?

A. 5%

B. 10%

C. 8%

D. 9%

15. Which of these fluids can be administered to a hypoglycemic neonate in the first 24 hours of life?

A. 10% dextrose water

B. Ringer's lactate

C. 4.3% dextrose saline

D. 5% dextrose saline

16. A child presents to the children's emergency room with signs and symptoms of intestinal obstruction. What electrolyte is at risk of depletion?

A. Sodium

B. Magnesium

C. Potassium

D. Chlorine

17. Which of the following is not a management option for hyperkalemia?

A. Insulin and dextrose infusion

B. Nebulized salbutamol

C. Resins

D. Calcium gluconate

18. Concerning type 1 diabetes mellitus, all of the following are true except ...

A. It is an autoimmune disease

B. Insulin is the drug of choice

C. There is destruction of the alpha cells in the pancreas

D. It is a childhood disease

19. A patient takes antidepressants to increase all of the following neurotransmitters except ...

A. Dopamine

B. Acetylcholine

C. Epinephrine

D. Serotonin

20. All of the following are possible features of peptic ulcer disease except ...

A. Melena stools

B. Epigastric pain

C. Hematemesis

D. Jaundice

21. A client with celiac disease has an intolerance to which of these foods?

A. Soy

B. Rye

C. Quinoa

D. Corn

22. A homeless alcoholic is most likely to be deficient in all of the following vitamins except ...

A. Folic acid

B. Thiamine

C. Ergosterol

D. Retinoic acid

23. A client who recently had gastric bypass surgery will be deficient in all of the following vitamins except ...

A. Iron

B. Zinc

C. Folate

D. Vitamin K

24. Which of the following interventions is appropriate for a client with end-stage hepatic failure?

A. Place on a high-protein diet

B. Give sedatives to relieve pain

C. Commence TPN

D. Monitor for constipation

25. All of the following clients are likely to present with melena stools except ...

A. A client with alcohol intoxication

B. A client with bulimia

C. A client on warfarin

D. A client with hemorrhoids

26. Concerning gynecomastia, which of the following is incorrect?

A. It's a precancerous state

B. Chronic kidney disease is a likely cause

C. It may be associated with galactorrhea

D. It is caused by an imbalance in the estrogen/androgen ratio

27. A female client complains of a thin, watery discharge with a characteristic fishy smell. She most likely has which of the following conditions?

A. Chlamydiosis

B. Candidiasis

C. Bacterial vaginosis

D. Herpes simplex

28. You are to give a health talk on cervical cancer to a group of parents, teachers and students in a high school. Which of the following information is correct?

A. Gardasil 9 prevents HPV 6, 8 and 18

B. Gardasil 9 should be given only to prepubertal girls

C. Gardasil 9 can be given to older people

D. Gardasil 9 offers protection from STIs

29. A couple presents to the clinic with infertility of three years. The wife has a history of induced abortion as a teenager. Which of the following is the correct diagnosis?

A. Primary infertility

B. Secondary infertility

C. Chronic PID

D. Hypogonadism

30. A woman with PCOS is least likely to have which of the following conditions or symptoms?

A. Infertility

B. Hirsutism

C. Diabetes

D. Unintentional weight loss

31. You are assessing the vital signs of an adult male client. Which of these vital signs is incorrectly matched to its functional diagnosis?

A. 39°C – hyperpyrexia

B. 30 cpm – tachypnea

C. 140/100 mmHg – hypertension

D. 100 bpm – tachycardia

32. All of the following are aseptic procedures except ...

A. Urethral catheterization

B. Venous catheterization

C. Colostomy irrigation

D. Umbilical catheterization

33. All of the following are correct about a nursing care plan except ...

A. It is used to define a nurse's role

B. It is constantly updated throughout a patient's admission

C. It can be formal or standardized

D. It is used to measure the quality of nursing care

34. Which of the following factors should be considered when admitting a male Muslim client to a ward?

A. The position of the bed

B. Type of fabric used for the bedsheets

C. The number of windows in the ward

D. Presence of handwashing sinks

35. Which of these foods is suitable for a Jewish American?

A. Shrimp salad with pasta

B. Yogurt, spaghetti and meatballs

C. Roasted chicken and vegetable fried rice

D. Bacon, scrambled eggs and a bagel

36. The following conversation ensues between a client with hypercholesterolemia and a nurse.

Client: Jogging is tiring for me—I find it difficult to breathe and my legs ache badly.

Nurse: Apart from jogging, what other milder exercises can you try?

What form of communication technology is this?

A. Giving advice

B. Forming a plan of action

C. Recognition

D. Giving false reassurances

37. A client says this to you: "I've been finding it difficult to sleep."

Which of the following examples describes the technique of placing an event in time or sequence?

A. When did this start?

B. How long do you sleep?

C. What do you eat before going to bed?

D. Do you get headaches?

38. A client involved in a road traffic accident says to you, “I shouldn’t have driven after drinking all that alcohol. I should have asked my friends to take me home.”

Which of these replies uses a therapeutic communication technique?

A. Next time, you will do the right thing.

B. It’s okay, you will make the right choices next time.

C. Why did you drink that amount of alcohol?

D. I see that you regret your actions.

39. A nurse tells a client with terminal cancer, “Don’t worry, you will feel better after the chemotherapy.”

This is an example of which communication technique?

A. Giving advice

B. Giving false reassurances

C. Defending

D. Giving approval

40. The following conversation ensues between a nurse and an anorexic client.

Client: I'm so fat. I need to control how I eat.

Nurse: Your BMI is 18 kg/m^2. You are underweight.

The nurse's reply is an example of which communication technique?

A. Making observations

B. Presenting reality

C. Giving advice

D. Recognition

41. Which of the following charges is handled by law enforcement?

A. Rude comments

B. Negligence

C. Malpractice

D. Health insurance fraud

42. Nurse E is charged with negligence of an epileptic patient. She will be held under what law?

A. Criminal

B. Civil

C. Administrative

D. Statutory

43. Decisions made by the state board of nursing fall under which of these laws?

A. Administrative law

B. Civil law

C. Common law

D. Criminal law

44. Which of the following types of nursing care for an obstetric client in labor can be done by a nursing assistant?

A. Vaginal examination

B. Blood pressure measurement

C. Monitor uterine contraction

D. Titrate oxytocin

45. A client has just had laparoscopic surgery for a ruptured ovarian cyst. Which of the following post-op care procedures is appropriate for an LPN?

A. Create a post-op nursing care plan

B. Administer IV antibiotics

C. Interpret hematological reports

D. Request a tissue biopsy

46. You are monitoring a client receiving a blood transfusion. You notice he starts showing symptoms of anaphylaxis. Which of the following is an appropriate first response?

A. Resuscitate the client with normal saline

B. Give intravenous corticosteroids

C. Stop the blood transfusion immediately

D. Give intravenous antibiotics

47. You are to give 1 g of IV Ceftriaxone to a client on admission. The client is currently on an IV infusion of Ringer's lactate. Which of the following is the most appropriate method to assess the compatibility of Ringer's lactate and Ceftriaxone?

A. Use a medication compatibility chart

B. Mix a small amount of the drug with a small amount of the fluid and observe for precipitates

C. Call the doctor and ask for compatibility

D. Mix a small amount of the drug with a small amount of the fluid and watch for color change

48. You are to give IM vitamin K to a 12-hour-old neonate. Which of these is the best site for administration?

A. Gluteus maximus

B. Vastus lateralis

C. Deltoid muscle

D. Biceps

49. A pediatric client with severe dehydration secondary to gastroenteritis will benefit from which of the following intravenous fluids?

A. 5% dextrose saline

B. 4.3% dextrose saline

C. 10% dextrose water

D. Ringer's lactate

50. A diabetic client presents to the emergency room with features of diabetic ketoacidosis (DKA). Which of the following intravenous fluids is used for acute resuscitation?

A. Ringer's lactate

B. Normal saline

C. Dextrose water

D. Dextrose saline

51. Concerning central lines, which of the following is correct?

A. A peripherally inserted central line is usually inserted in the subclavian vein

B. Centrally non-tunneled central lines are also called Hickman Lines

C. Implantable ports are required for obese patients with invisible veins

D. Implantable ports are not indicated for cachectic and obese patients

52. A client presents to the emergency room with dizziness, rashes on the trunk and arms and swelling of his lips and both eyelids. A history of recent NSAID use is obtained. This patient will benefit from the immediate actions of all the following drugs except ...

A. Omalizumab

B. IV epinephrine

C. IV hydrocortisone

D. Nebulized salbutamol

53. Your client is taking isoniazid as part of his regimen for HIV. He is at risk of having which of the following deficiencies?

A. Pyridoxine

B. Riboflavin

C. Cobalamin

D. Niacin

54. All the following drugs are likely causes of drug-induced paresthesia except ...

A. Nitrofurantoin

B. Isoniazid

C. Cobalamin supplements

D. Phenytoin

55. Which of the following is a WHO principle of pain management?

A. Step 1 involves the use of oxycodone with or without adjuvants

B. Step 1 involves the use of diclofenac with or without adjuvants

C. Step 1 involves the use of prednisolone with or without adjuvants

D. Step 1 involves the use of diazepam with or without adjuvants

56. Which of the following is a weak opioid?

A. Fentanyl

B. Methadone

C. Hydrocodone

D. Oxycodone

57. Concerning Naltrexone, which of the following is correct?

A. It is an opioid agonist

B. It is an opioid antagonist

C. It is indicated in acetaminophen overdose

D. Side effects include diarrhea

58. A preterm neonate with RDS will benefit from a surfactant given through which of the following routes?

A. Intradermal

B. Subcutaneous

C. Intratracheal

D. Intravenous

59. Estrogen therapy will be beneficial to all of the following clients except ...

A. A 58-year-old woman with fibroids

B. A 22-year-old college student with dysfunctional uterine bleeding

C. A 75-year-old woman with hot flushes

D. A 30-year-old woman with primary hypogonadism

60. A six-year-old male with a respiratory rate of 30 cpm has ...

A. A fast respiratory rate

B. A normal respiratory rate

C. A slow respiratory rate

D. Bilateral crepitations

61. A pediatric client presents to the emergency room with a cough, fast breathing, fever and snoring. As the nurse on duty, you will need to examine the child's tonsils using all of the following except ...

A. A pen flashlight

B. A laryngoscope

C. A spatula

D. A swab stick

62. Which of the following clients has the greatest risk of deep vein thrombosis?

A. A primigravida with twin gestation

B. A female client on estrogen replacement therapy

C. A male client with a history of smoking five packs a day for years

D. A client who has undergone hip replacement surgery

63. A hypertensive client presents to the emergency room with complaints of sudden onset of chest pain and difficulty breathing. All of the following enzymes can be used for myocardial indication except ...

A. Troponin

B. ALP

C. CK MB

D. LDH

E. Myoglobin

64. Which of the following clients has the greatest risk for orthostatic pneumonia?

A. A client with recurrent GERD

B. A client with esophageal candidiasis

C. An elderly client with metastatic CAP to the lumbar vertebrae

D. A client with a laryngeal tumor

65. All of the following causes of jaundice can be managed with phototherapy except ...

A. Neonatal sepsis

B. Cephalohematoma

C. Polycythemia

D. Dubin–Johnson Syndrome

66. Which of the following is not a feature of pathologic jaundice in a newborn?

A. Jaundice from the fourth day of life

B. Jaundice that lasts more than two weeks

C. Jaundice with associated fever

D. Jaundice with rapidly rising levels

67. All the following can be used to assess a child's dehydration status except ...

A. Skin turgidity

B. Buccal mucosa

C. Capillary refill

D. Respiratory rate

68. All of the following can be used to assess pallor except ...

A. The palmar surfaces of the hands and feet

B. Conjunctiva

C. Buccal mucosa

D. Sclera

69. A client with a platelet count of 100,000 mcL will likely present with which of the following signs?

A. Petechiae rash

B. Erythema

C. Malar rash

D. Miliaria

70. All of the following are possible complications of an obese patient who has just had gastric bypass surgery except ...

A. Impaired wound healing

B. Deep vein thrombosis

C. Orthostatic pneumonia

D. Wound dehiscence

71. A client with a total protein of 5.5 g/dL is at risk for all of the following except …

A. Ascites

B. Impaired wound healing

C. Urolithiasis

D. Pitting edema

72. Which of the following methods is employed to reduce muscle atrophy in a bedridden patient?

A. Give calcium supplements

B. Provide muscle physiotherapy

C. Feed a protein-rich diet

D. Give iron supplements

73. Nursing care for a bedridden patient includes which of the following?

A. Using linen layers to minimize soiling

B. Performing skin assessments every two days using the Braden scale

C. Turning the client from left, right and back every two hours to relieve pressure

D. Lubricating pressure points with petroleum jelly to reduce friction

74. A client with GERD complains of a burning sensation in the epigastric region. This client will get instant relief if placed in which of the following positions?

A. High Fowler's position

B. Low Fowler's position

C. Lithotomy position

D. Reverse Trendelenburg position

75. A two-month-old female with a cleft palate may have any of the following feeding challenges except ...

A. Aspiration

B. Malabsorption

C. Dental caries

D. Regurgitation

76. Which of the following clients will benefit from being placed in a semi-Fowler's position?

A. A client who had a craniotomy for cerebral hemorrhage

B. A client who had a herniorrhaphy

C. A client who had spinal anesthesia

D. A client who had a laparoscopic liver biopsy

77. Which of the following clients will not benefit from having a limb elevated?

A. A client with post-op amputation of the left leg

B. A client who is one hour post-op from an arterio-vascular graft

C. A client with pedal edema secondary to right heart failure

D. A client with deep venous thrombosis

78. You are counseling your client with GERD on how to find relief from symptoms of bloating and heartburn. Which of the following guidelines is incorrect?

A. Eat small, frequent meals

B. Eat highly fatty foods to improve bile secretion

C. Eat fewer citrus fruits

D. Stay in an upright position for 30 minutes after eating

79. Which of the following conditions is incorrectly matched to its nursing intervention?

A. Constipation – enema

B. Pyrexia – cold water baths

C. Laryngectomy – semi-Fowler's position

D. DVT – limb elevation

80. You have a terminally ill client with advanced prostatic cancer. Although he has been told of the outcome of his condition, he carries on with making plans for a trip to the Swiss Alps as soon as he is discharged from the hospital. What defense mechanism is the client utilizing?

A. Suppression

B. Denial

C. Reaction formation

D. Regression

81. A client being managed for conduct disorder insists that he acts the way he does because no one likes him. What defense mechanism is the client engaging in?

A. Introjection

B. Projection

C. Sublimation

D. Repression

82. Which of these models identifies attitudes, bias and systemic barriers that make it difficult for people with an impairment to function well?

A. Social model of disability

B. Biomedical model of disability

C. Cognitive model of disability

D. Biosocial model of disability

83. Which of the following principles is correct concerning the biomedical model of disability?

A. Treating and managing disabilities

B. Methods and principles of early intervention to prevent disability

C. A focus on environmental and social exclusions

D. The basis of the social model of disability

84. A six-month-old client presents to the pediatric clinic for routine immunization. You expect the client to have achieved which of the following developmental milestones?

A. Responding to his own name

B. Following simple instructions

C. Standing with support

D. Making a two-to-four-word sentence

85. Ana is a two-year-old toddler. You expect Ana to have achieved all the following milestones except ...

A. Following simple instructions

B. Pointing to things in a book

C. Building a tower of two or more blocks

D. Telling stories

86. Which of the following clients is most vulnerable to elder abuse?

A. A 65-year-old male with osteoarthritis

B. A 70-year-old male with prostate cancer

C. A 75-year-old female with Alzheimer's disease

D. A 59-year-old female with advanced cervical cancer

87. You are assessing a day-old neonate born at 32 weeks gestation. You expect all of the following physical characteristics except ...

A. Lanugo hair

B. Overgrown nails

C. A disproportionately large head

D. Shiny pink skin

88. You are to auscultate the lung fields of a client with COPD. Which of the following is correct?

A. Diminished vesicular breath sounds can indicate COPD

B. Bronchial breath sounds are normal breath sounds

C. Breath sounds are loudest at the base in early inspiration

D. Breath sounds are loudest at the apex in mid-inspiration

89. You are auscultating the heart sounds of a client. Which of the following is correct?

A. S1 and S2 are both loud in the cardiac area

B. S1 is faint at the apex and S2 is loud at the base

C. S1 is loud at the apex and S2 is faint at the base

D. S1 is loud at the apex and S2 is loud at the base

90. A client with decompensated liver disease is most likely to have which of the following?

A. A positive fluid thrill

B. A negative fluid thrill

C. A negative shifting dullness

D. A positive Kernig's sign

91. Ballotable kidneys can indicate which of the following?

A. A horseshoe kidney

B. Contracted kidneys

C. Hydronephrosis

D. Renal hypoplasia

92. You are to give a handwashing demonstration to a group of fourth-grade kids. Which of the following guidelines is incorrect?

A. Scrub your hands for at least 10 seconds

B. Wash your hands before eating food

C. Wash your hands after using the toilet

D. Use a sanitizer that contains at least 60% alcohol

93. Which of the following vaccines is correctly matched to its corresponding schedule?

A. DPT – 12 weeks

B. Rotavirus – 10 weeks

C. Hepatitis B – from birth

D. PCV – 4 weeks

94. Which of the following is not a conjugate vaccine?

A. Pertussis vaccine

B. Hepatitis B vaccine

C. HPV vaccine

D. Tetanus vaccine

95. A day-old neonate born at 30 weeks is at risk for all of the following complications except ...

A. Respiratory distress

B. Polycythemia

C. NEC

D. PDA

96. Breast milk's easy digestibility makes it the recommended food for infants. Which of the following factors contributes to breast milk digestibility?

A. A high casein content

B. A high whey content

C. Bifidus factor

D. IgA

97. Which of the following clients is ineligible for a rotavirus vaccine?

A. A 4-year-old female with hemophilia

B. A 5-year-old male with a history of intussusception

C. A 30-year-old male with HIV

D. A 15-year-old teenager with type 1 diabetes mellitus

98. A neonate born at 30 weeks will benefit from kangaroo mother care. All of the following are benefits of kangaroo mother care except ...

A. Breastfeeding

B. Warmth

C. Bonding

D. Phototherapy

99. Which of the following is a preventive measure for hepatitis A?

A. Avoid sharing of spoons and plates

B. Handwashing

C. Avoid sharing of sharps and needles

D. Avoid direct contact with bloodstained bedding

100. Which of the following best explains the pathophysiology of pruritus in obstructive jaundice?

A. Impaired urea excretion

B. Impaired bile acid absorption

C. Impaired metabolism of bilirubin

D. Impaired bile acid excretion

Test 3

1. A 12-hour-old neonate born with a birth weight of 5 kg is at risk of all of the following complications except ...

A. Hypoglycemia

B. Cephalohematoma

C. Birth asphyxia

D. Hypothermia

2. A client is contemplating the use of a copper IUD for contraception and seeks your expert advice. All of the following are possible risk factors associated with copper IUDs except ...

A. Pelvic inflammatory disease

B. Menorrhagia

C. Perforation

D. Weight gain

3. All of the following breast milk properties are accurately matched to their uses except ...

A. High whey content – easy digestibility

B. Lactoferrin – inhibits the growth of iron-dependent bacteria

C. IgA – supports the growth of lactobacillus

D. DHEA – improves cognition

4. A component of newborn care is administering antibiotic ointments into the eyes within two hours after birth to prevent conjunctivitis. Which of the following microbes is susceptible to the antibiotics?

A. Chlamydia

B. Herpes

C. Syphilis

D. E. coli

5. A gravid client at 20 weeks gestation has an FBS of 6.1 mmol/L. This client is at risk of developing all of the following complications except ...

A. Spontaneous abortion

B. Obstructed labor

C. Preeclampsia

D. Neonatal jaundice

6. Which of the following communicable diseases is not preventable through handwashing?

A. Scabies

B. Cholera

C. Flu

D. Meningitis

7. A 7-year-old client is currently being treated for scabies. Which of the following is a primary prevention method to reduce the risk of spread to other members of the child's family?

A. Dispose of all used clothes and underwear

B. Wash hands frequently with antiseptic soap

C. Wash and store all clothes in airtight bags for at least 48 hours

D. Immunize all family members with the scabies vaccine

8. All of the following are preventable causes of first trimester miscarriages except ...

A. TORCHES infection

B. Diabetes mellitus

C. Cervical insufficiency

D. Ionizing radiation

9. Your client, who has a history of chronic nicotine use, says he can't stop smoking cigarettes because whenever he does, he has nausea and vomiting. Which of the following statements is correct?

A. This client has a psychological dependence on nicotine use

B. This client has a physical dependence on nicotine use

C. This client is suffering from nicotine overdose

D. This client has a cognitive dependence on nicotine

10. A client with acrophobia will benefit from which of the following psychotherapy interventions?

A. Family therapy

B. Aversive conditioning

C. Systemic desensitization

D. Psychoanalysis

11. A client with personality disorders will benefit from which of the following psychotherapy interventions?

A. Family therapy

B. Group therapy

C. Behavioral therapy

D. Aversive conditioning

12. You are interacting with a teenage client in the pediatric clinic. All of the following are traits peculiar to teenagers except ...

A. Concrete thinking

B. Independence

C. Risk-taking

D. Solitude

13. An anorexic client presents to the emergency unit. Which of the following interventions should be prioritized?

A. Start the client on TPN

B. Start the client on intravenous dextrose infusion

C. Start the client on a psychotherapy intervention

D. Monitor vital signs, electrolytes and blood gases

14. A couple presents to the children's emergency room with their injured two-year-old child. All of the following features point to a likely case of child abuse except ...

A. Injuries are inconsistent with the behavior and age of the child

B. The child remains silent during the physical examination

C. The child refuses to make eye contact with the examiner

D. The parents give conflicting histories

15. Your client has just been diagnosed with child abuse, which his parents perpetrated. Which of the following interventions should be prioritized?

A. Explore the family dynamics involved

B. Sedate the child

C. Ensure the safety of the child

D. Discuss the implications of child abuse with the parents

16. An autistic child will benefit from which of the following social environments?

A. An environment that is familiar and routine

B. An environment that is safe and diverse

C. An environment that is accepting and spontaneous

D. An environment that is secure and colorful

17. You notice that your bedridden client has developed sacral pressure ulcers. These ulcers are fresh, with a red base. All of the following interventions are correct except ...

A. Covering the ulcer's surface with a hydrocolloid film

B. Using cotton sheets to minimize shearing

C. Turning the client every two hours

D. Debriding the wound with a surgical laser

18. Your client on nasogastric feeding will benefit from which of the following interventions?

A. Increasing fiber intake to prevent constipation

B. Increasing water intake to prevent urinary tract infection

C. Maintaining a slow infusion rate to prevent overfeeding and diarrhea

D. Daily turning of the client

19. A client undergoing chemotherapy will benefit from all of the following interventions except ...

A. Antiemetics for nausea and vomiting

B. Adequate water intake to prevent urolithiasis

C. Adequate analgesia for chronic pain

D. High-protein diet to prevent muscle atrophy

20. Your client undergoing chemotherapy has nausea and a subsequent loss of appetite. Which of the following nursing interventions will be beneficial?

A. Insert a nasogastric tube

B. Start the client on intravenous 10% dextrose water infusion

C. Encourage the client to eat small, frequent meals

D. Encourage the client to eat spicy foods

21. All of the following are management guidelines for a client with a tracheostomy except ...

A. Provide a bell, pen and paper

B. Tracheostomy changes are done daily or when soiled with secretions

C. Remove old ties before securing new ones

D. A minimum of two people are required for a tie change

22. Your client is scheduled to have a liver biopsy tomorrow for suspected liver cirrhosis. She is unable to sleep and complains of headaches and palpitations. Which of the following is an appropriate nursing intervention?

A. Give a sedative

B. Inform the psychiatrist

C. Encourage the client to meditate and visualize

D. Use a therapeutic communication technique

23. A two-year-old child is scheduled for surgery under general anesthesia. If the surgery is scheduled for 8 a.m. the next day, which of the following fasting options will be most comfortable for the child?

A. Overnight fast from 10 p.m.

B. Stop solid food by 10 p.m., then the child can drink breast milk till 6 a.m.

C. Stop solid food by 12 a.m., then the child can drink breast milk till 2 a.m. and can drink clear fluids till 6 a.m.

D. Stop solid food from 12 a.m., then the child can drink clear fluids till 7 a.m.

24. A year-old client scheduled for a tonsillectomy can drink all of the following fluids two hours before surgery except ...

A. Water

B. Apple juice

C. Yogurt

D. Pedialyte

25. Hartmann's solution is not indicated in which of the following conditions?

A. Acute intestinal obstruction

B. 30% burns

C. End-stage renal disease

D. Acute pancreatitis

26. Calculate the drop rate of a 500-ml IV fluid that should be administered over eight hours via an intravenous set that delivers 20 gtt/ml.

A. 11 gtt/min

B. 22 gtt/min

C. 21 gtt/min

D. 13 gtt/min

27. A neonate is to receive 150 ml of dextrose water over six hours using a soluset. What is the drop rate?

A. 20 gtt/min

B. 25 gtt/min

C. 30 gtt/min

D. 15 gtt/min

28. Which of the following is the ideal route of administration for vancomycin?

A. As an intravenous bolus

B. As an intravenous infusion

C. As an intramuscular bolus

D. As an oral suspension

29. Which of the following side effects is correctly matched to its corresponding drug?

A. Streptomycin – paresthesia

B. Tetracycline – gum discoloration

C. Isoniazid – deafness

D. Metronidazole – diarrhea

30. Which of the following cannulae is appropriate for an obstetric client in labor?

A. 18G

B. 20G

C. 22G

D. 24G

31. Oxytocin use is indicated in all of the following conditions except ...

A. Post-term pregnancy

B. Miscarriage

C. Preeclampsia

D. Placenta previa

32. All of the following drugs have vomiting as a side effect except ...

A. Epirubicin

B. Methotrexate

C. Paclitaxel

D. Ondansetron

33. A woman in preterm labor will benefit from all of the following except ...

A. Salbutamol

B. Magnesium sulfate

C. Ergometrine

D. Dexamethasone

34. Which of the following drugs is unlikely to cause Stevens–Johnson syndrome?

A. Nevirapine

B. Allopurinol

C. Acetazolamide

D. Chloroquine

35. All of the following are valuable tools for assessing pain in an adult except ...

A. McGill-Melzack pain questionnaire

B. Simple description pain intensity scale

C. Faces pain rating scale

D. 0–10 numeric pain scale

36. Which of the following is least likely to cause an albumin of 2.5 g/dL?

A. Liver cirrhosis

B. Nephrotic syndrome

C. Diabetes mellitus

D. Malabsorption syndrome

37. A client presents to the emergency unit with complaints of headaches, blurry vision and chest pain. His blood pressure is 170/120 mmHg. This client is at risk of all of the following complications except ...

A. Stroke

B. Myocardial infarction

C. Papillary edema

D. Thrombocytopenia

38. A client on maintenance therapy for warfarin has a prothrombin time of 25 seconds. Based on this result, which of the following actions is necessary?

A. Withhold the next dose of warfarin

B. Increase the next dose of warfarin

C. Give the next dose of warfarin

D. Decrease the next dose of warfarin

39. A primigravida at 16 weeks is scheduled to have an alpha-fetoprotein test. Which of the following is true?

A. This test is diagnostic of chromosomal disorders

B. This test is diagnostic of lung anomalies

C. This test is diagnostic of neural tube defects

D. This test is diagnostic of cardiac defects

40. A bedridden client is at risk of all of the following except ...

A. Pressure ulcers

B. Hypercalcemia

C. Orthostatic pneumonia

D. Diarrhea

41. A female client who complains of a sudden attack of severe pain, swelling, redness and tenderness of the joints has a uric acid level of 8 mg/dL. Which of the following statements is incorrect?

A. This client has rheumatoid arthritis

B. Obesity is a risk factor

C. She should substitute red meat with seafood

D. Alcohol consumption is a risk factor

42. A known ESRD patient presents to the emergency unit with unconsciousness and deep apneic breathing. His electrolyte results are as follows:

Sodium – 130 mmol/L

Potassium – 5.7 mmol/L

Urea – 35 mmol/L

Creatinine – 400 umol/L

Bicarbonate – 15 mmol/L

This client has which of the following conditions?

A. Respiratory acidosis

B. Metabolic alkaloids

C. Respiratory alkalosis

D. Metabolic acidosis

43. A female client with known anxiety disorder presents to the emergency room with fast breathing, palpitations and chest pain following an unsuccessful job interview. Her arterial blood gases are as follows:

HCO_3 – 25 mmol/L

pH – 7.6

PCO_2 – 20 mmHg.

This client has ...

A. Metabolic acidosis

B. Respiratory acidosis

C. Metabolic alkaloid

D. Respiratory alkalosis

44. All of the following are absolute indications for a caesarean section except ...

A. Two or more previous caesarean sections

B. Twin gestation

C. Previous myomectomy

D. Cephalopelvic disproportion

45. Which of the following is the accurate measurement of a feeding tube?

A. From the tip of the nose to the earlobe to the xiphisternum

B. From the tip of the nose to the chin to the xiphisternum

C. From the tip of the nose to the earlobe to the sternum

D. From the tip of the nose to the pinna to the xiphisternum

46. A client has a chest tube inserted for massive pleural effusion. The nurse notices the continuous bubbling of the suction control of the chamber. Which of the following interpretations is correct?

A. There is a possible air leak

B. The chest tube is draining actively

C. The chest tube is dislodged from the pleura space

D. The suction pressure is reduced

47. Which of the following clients will not benefit from an elevated head of the bed position?

A. A client with a laryngectomy

B. A client with cerebral edema

C. A client with a pleural effusion

D. A client with a lumbar puncture

48. A patient with CVD has aphasia. Which of the following lobes of the cerebral cortex is affected?

A. Occipital lobe

B. Frontal lobe

C. Parietal lobe

D. Sagittal lobe

49. Which of the following GCS scores is indicative of a severe head injury?

A. 12

B. 4

C. 9

D. 15

50. A client presents to the emergency unit with opioid overdose. On GCS examination there was no eye opening. The client had an extension response to pain and made incomprehensible sounds. What is this client's GCS score?

A. 6

B. 5

C. 3

D. 4

51. Benefits of gut flora include all of the following except ...

A. Vitamin K synthesis

B. Carbohydrate metabolism

C. Vitamin C metabolism

D. Vitamin B12 metabolism

52. A hypertensive female client will benefit from which of the following family planning methods?

A. Copper IUD

B. Low-dose pills

C. Bilateral tubal ligation

D. COCP

53. A female client with hyperprolactinemia will most likely complain of all of the following except ...

A. Galactorrhea

B. Headaches

C. Infertility

D. Increased libido

54. A female client with recurrent UTIs will be advised to do all of the following except ...

A. Use prophylactic antibiotics

B. Observe good wiping hygiene

C. Wear nylon underwear

D. Increase water intake

55. A male client with left pleural effusion is expected to have which of the following?

A. Resonant percussion notes on the left anterior chest wall

B. Dull percussion notes on the left anterior chest wall

C. Stony dull percussion notes on the left anterior chest wall

D. Tympanic percussion notes on the left anterior chest wall

56. A client with an inflammation of the right lung lobe is expected to have which of the following?

A. Resonant percussion notes on the right anterior chest wall

B. Dull percussion notes on the right anterior chest wall

C. Stony dull percussion notes on the right anterior chest wall

D. Tympanic percussion notes on the right anterior chest wall

57. When passing a nasogastric tube, which of the following methods confirms the tube is in the trachea?

A. Presence of bubbles when the free end of the tube is placed in water

B. Aspiration of green fluid

C. Vesicular breath sounds on auscultation

D. Stony dull percussion notes of the chest wall

58. Cigarette smoke can trigger pneumonia via which of the following pathologic processes?

A. Inflammation

B. Metabolic derangement

C. Hemolysis

D. Degeneration

59. An asthmatic is not likely to have which of the following pathophysiologic responses?

A. Increased mucus production

B. Bronchiolar hypertrophy

C. Airway narrowing

D. Increased mucociliary action

60. All of the following are likely features of a blue bloater except ...

A. Cyanosis

B. Peripheral edema

C. Barrel-shaped chest

D. Obesity

61. All of the following are likely features of a pink puffer except ...

A. Pink skin

B. Chronic productive cough

C. Cachectic appearance

D. Pursed lip breathing

62. Which of the following is least likely to cause respiratory acidosis?

A. Myasthenia gravis

B. Diabetic ketoacidosis

C. Chronic bronchitis

D. Emphysema

63. All of the following are possible complications of community-acquired lobar pneumonia in children except ...

A. Acute heart failure

B. Pericarditis

C. Septic shock

D. Pott's Disease

64. A client with nephrotic syndrome is unlikely to have hypertension because ...

A. There is a loss of protein and salt

B. Fluid retention is not in the vascular space

C. There is increased plasma oncotic pressure

D. There is increased plasma hydrostatic pressure

65. All of the following waste materials must be disposed of in the black waste container except ...

A. Cytotoxic drugs

B. Expired drugs

C. Blood bags

D. Radioactive substances

66. When disposing of used sharps, which of the following guidelines is incorrect?

A. Cap used needles before disposal

B. Dispose of used needles in the sharps container

C. The sharps container is not used to dispose of syringes

D. Sharps containers should be tightly sealed

67. A 5-year-old child who has scabies has transmitted the infestation to her younger siblings. Which of the following was the most likely route of transmission?

A. Swimming in the same pool

B. Poor cough etiquette

C. Sleeping in the same bed

D. Eating from the same plate

68. A new mother needs counseling on feeding options for her infant. Which of the following guidelines is correct?

A. Commence solid foods from five months

B. Breastfeed exclusively with breast milk for nine months

C. Give vitamin D-fortified cow's milk when the child is one year

D. Breastfeed baby for at least two years

69. You are to provide contraceptives to a client. Which of the following guidelines is correct?

A. Use progesterone-only contraceptives to reduce the risk of cervical cancer

B. Use COCP to increase compliance

C. Add a barrier contraceptive to prevent STI transmission

D. Use a copper IUD if the client has multiple sexual partners

70. A client has a serum potassium of 6.5 mmol/L. Which of the following is given to increase the threshold potential of the cardiac cells and reduce the risk of ventricular fibrillation?

A. Calcium chloride

B. Salbutamol

C. Insulin

D. Hartmann's solution

71. A gravid client has an FBS result of 6 mmol/L. Which of the following guidelines is appropriate in managing her condition?

A. Diet modification and aerobic exercise

B. Use of insulin and metformin

C. Use of metformin only

D. Use of insulin only

72. A client presents to the clinic with an occupational health disease. Which of the following guidelines is accurate concerning the management of this client?

A. Laboratory tests for target organs are usually specific for making a diagnosis

B. Remove the client from the workplace before commencing management

C. Exposure to an agent at a level below legal occupational exposure limits excludes the possibility of an occupational health disease

D. Inquiries should be made about similar symptoms in colleagues and coworkers

73. Which of the following hazards is incorrectly matched to its example?

A. Biological hazard – needle-prick injuries

B. Chemical hazards – mercury poisoning

C. Physical hazard – sexual harassment at work

D. Ergonomic hazard – slouching at work desks

74. You are to give a public health presentation to a group of cooks at a high school. Which of the following is not a component of food safety?

A. Wash hands, utensils and work surfaces

B. Separate raw food from cooked food

C. Serve all food hot

D. Store food at the proper temperature

75. Concerning gloves, which of the following is incorrect?

A. Non-sterile gloves are safe for touching mucous membranes

B. Non-sterile gloves are safe for performing septic procedures

C. Non-sterile gloves are used for handling infectious materials

D. You should change gloves when moving from a contaminated area to a non-contaminated area

76. Concerning airborne isolation guidelines, which of the following is correct?

A. Disease-causing microbes are suspended in the air as particles and aerosols

B. Infected clients should be isolated in negative pressure rooms

C. Infected clients should be isolated in positive pressure rooms

D. Disposable N95 masks are used only to cover the nose

77. You are to supervise a newly licensed RN who is working her first shift in the emergency room. Which of the following clients is suitable for this RN?

A. A 70-year-old client with HHS

B. A 23-year-old client with a closed fracture of the right humerus

C. A 20-year-old client with opioid overdose

D. A 25-year-old client with a dislocated ankle

78. You are supervising an LPN who is teaching a diabetic client how to use a glucometer. Which of the following steps is incorrect?

A. Swab the finger with an alcohol rub

B. Turn on the glucometer and insert a strip into the machine

C. When the indicator turns on, pierce the pad of the finger

D. Place the drop of blood on the strip

79. A client is treated for SIADH. Serial monitoring is needed for which of the following electrolytes?

A. Sodium

B. Potassium

C. Chlorine

D. Bicarbonate

80. A client's ECG is shown to have inverted T waves and prominent U waves. Which of the following electrolytes is implicated?

A. Sodium

B. Potassium

C. Calcium

D. Chlorine

81. You are responsible for a client with ESRD. Which of the following nursing care interventions can be supervised by a nursing assistant?

A. Alternate-day weighing

B. Serial electrolyte monitoring

C. Planning a restricted protein diet

D. Assisting clients with feeding

82. Priorities are important in helping nurses anticipate and organize multiple nursing interventions. These priorities are determined by which of the following?

A. The client's socioeconomic status

B. Urgency of need

C. The ordering physician

D. The client's family

83. Patient-centered care allows clients to participate in their own management. In order for the client to participate, he/she must be ...

A. Alert and capacitated

B. Literate

C. Ambulatory

D. Financially sound

84. RNs rank higher than nursing assistants and LPNs. Which of the following reasons best explains why?

A. They earn more money

B. Their education is more expensive

C. They are natural leaders

D. They are more proficient in the required knowledge, education and skills

85. Which of the following best describes a nursing care plan?

A. A document that contains information about a client's diagnosis and goal of treatment

B. A document that is created by the most senior nurse on a team

C. A uniform template used for all clients

D. A legal document signed by the American Nurses Association

86. All of the following are parts of the nursing process except ...

A. Assessment

B. Planning

C. Treatment

D. Evaluation

87. In the delivery room, your client desires that nobody make a sound when the baby is born until her husband whispers a prayer in the baby's ear. Your client practices which of the following religions?

A. Islam

B. Christianity

C. Hinduism

D. Judaism

88. Which of the following religions is least likely to consent to organ donation after death?

A. Jehovah's Witness

B. Shinto

C. Judaism

D. Presbyterianism

89. A Chinese client is brought to the emergency room with acute hemorrhage from a ruptured ectopic pregnancy. After recovery, the client believes she has a Yang disorder. Which of the following meals will she recommend for herself?

A. Hot tea

B. Ice water

C. Frozen yogurt

D. Salad

90. Which of the following religions is tolerant of cremation?

A. Islam

B. Christianity

C. Judaism

D. Hinduism

91. All of the following are examples of therapeutic communication techniques except ...

A. Reflection

B. Restating

C. Paraphrasing

D. Probing

92. All of the following are examples of quantitative research except ...

A. Correlational research

B. Descriptive research

C. Ethnographic research

D. Quasi-experimental research

93. Which of the following is a primary source for research data?

A. Articles

B. Book reviews

C. Journals

D. Surveys

94. Which of the following is not a secondary source of data?

A. Video and audio recordings

B. Book reviews

C. Journal critiques

D. Newspaper clippings

95. Which of the following is true concerning an experimental research study?

A. It is a qualitative research design

B. This design identifies people without participation and interference

C. It uses open-ended questions to generate qualitative data

D. It is conducted with a scientific approach to assess quantitative data

96. All of the following are qualities of a hypothesis except ...

A. Measurable

B. Testable

C. Abstract

D. Contains a variable

97. All of the following are clinical features found in a preeclamptic patient except ...

A. Pedal edema

B. Proteinuria

C. Blurred vision

D. Headaches

98. In assessing a patient with acute hemorrhage, which of the following signs is least likely on examination?

A. Bradycardia

B. Normotension

C. Tachycardia

D. Tachypnea

99. A female patient is admitted to the emergency unit with lower abdominal pain and profuse vaginal bleeding from a suspected cervical malignancy. The top nursing goal is which of the following?

A. Alleviate pain

B. Do a cervical examination to assess bleeding

C. Treat underlying infection

D. Resuscitate with isotonic fluids

100. A pregnant client comes for her first ANC visit. Her obstetric history includes a 5-year-old male who is alive, a term stillbirth three years ago and two miscarriages at 10 and 16 weeks. Which of the following accurately captures this information?

A. Gravida 5 para 4

B. Gravida 5 para 2

C. Gravida 3 para 2

D. Gravida 3 para 4

Test 4

1. You are conducting a study to determine whether shorter hospital admissions reduce the risk of nosocomial MRSA infection. What kind of a variable is the phrase “shorter hospital admissions”?

A. Dependent variable

B. Independent variable

C. Control variable

D. Responding variable

2. What kind of a variable is the phrase “risk of nosocomial MRSA infection”?

A. Dependent variable

B. Control variable

C. Independent variable

D. Constant variable

3. Which of the following is correct about the functional nursing model?

A. It is task-oriented

B. It is client-oriented

C. Clients are assigned tasks to make them more involved

D. It encourages a client-nurse relationship

4. Which of the following is not a feature of a decentralized organizational structure?

A. Tall structure

B. Bottom-up philosophy

C. Delegation

D. Autonomy

5. Nurse G. knows how to communicate with her team members. As a team leader, she inspires her members to get things done. Her team members are motivated by her personality and energy. What kind of leader is Nurse G?

A. Transformational

B. Visionary

C. Charismatic

D. Reactionary

6. All of the following are features of a centralized workplace except ...

A. Tall structure

B. Top-to-bottom model

C. Hierarchal

D. Autonomy

7. Nurse M is very interested in the future of the hospital. He encourages his team members by constantly reminding them of the vision and potential of the hospital. However, as a leader, he is open to suggestions that can help the team achieve the vision. What kind of leader is Nurse M?

A. Transformational

B. Charismatic

C. Visionary

D. Democratic

8. Nurse A is assigned to organize the new pediatric ward in the hospital. She designs a structure that allows communication and feedback to flow to two separate chains of command. What form of organizational structure is this?

A. Centralized

B. Informal

C. Cubical

D. Matrix

9. Nurse A later decides to redesign the ward in a way that allows information and feedback to flow in all directions. This feature is characteristic of which organizational structure?

A. Decentralized

B. Modular

C. Matrix

D. Centralized

10. All of the following are uses of qualitative research methods except ...

A. Creating survey instruments

B. Developing a theory

C. Creating clinical guidelines

D. Studying outcomes on a variable

11. Which of the following best describes the difference between qualitative and quantitative research?

A. Qualitative research is used for textual data, while quantitative research is used for numerical data

B. Qualitative research is used to create a hypothesis for phenomena, while quantitative research is used to explore phenomena

C. Qualitative research has a stable study design, while quantitative research has a flexible design

D. Qualitative research uses structured techniques, while quantitative research uses unstructured and semi-structured techniques

12. Which of the following meals is suitable for a devout Hindu patient?

A. Chicken salad and pasta

B. Tofu salad with basmati rice

C. Lamb curry with rice

D. Hamburger and milkshake

13. Which of the following clients is most at risk for developing hypertension?

A. A 35 year old Indian American

B. A 49-year-old African American

C. A 55-year-old Japanese American

D. A 25-year-old Jewish American

14. Which of the following is an open-ended question?

A. Do you exercise regularly?

B. What do you think about making aerobic exercise part of your weekly routine?

C. Are you doing enough exercise?

D. Can you eat more fruits and fewer carbohydrates?

15. The following conversation ensues between a nurse and a client who is being prepped for surgery.

Client: For the last two days, I have woken up at 3 a.m. and found myself unable to go back to sleep.

Which of the following responses is a general lead technique?

A. I see

B. Okay

C. I'm listening

D. You are probably anxious about brain surgery

16. Which of the following communication techniques acknowledges a patient's behavior without giving compliments, flattery or approval?

A. Making observation

B. Giving recognition

C. Paraphrasing

D. Giving false reassurance

17. The following conversation ensues between a client with severe depression and a nurse.

Client: I don't think I can carry on anymore. I'm so tired of feeling like this.

Nurse: You need to start focusing on positive thoughts.

The nurse's response is an example of which communication technique?

A. Presenting reality

B. Making observation

C. Recognition

D. Giving advice

18. A teenage client being managed for an STI confesses that she has multiple sexual partners. She says, “I don’t believe in love. Love is overrated.” Which of the following responses uses a therapeutic communication technique?

A. Love and commitment are necessary for any relationship

B. You are putting yourself at risk for cervical cancer and HIV

C. Don’t you think you are too young to have sex?

D. I see you don’t trust people easily

19. You come in contact with a new mother who has refused to vaccinate her two-week-old infant. She says vaccines make children autistic. Which of these responses uses a therapeutic technique?

A. Your theory is incorrect and controversial

B. You are putting your baby at risk of infectious diseases

C. You don’t have a good health education

D. I see you are afraid of vaccines

20. A client who exercises his right to refuse treatment is protected by which of the following laws?

A. Civil law

B. Common law

C. Criminal law

D. Statutory law

21. Which of the following describes a document that allows a guarantor to act on behalf of someone who is unable to act for himself?

A. An advance directive

B. A living will

C. A durable power of attorney

D. Informed consent

22. Which of the following is incorrect about informed consent?

A. It is written permission granted by a client to a doctor for medical treatment, after being made aware of the risks and benefits

B. It is not used for illiterate clients

C. It is done voluntarily

D. Informed consent can be given by proxy

23. All of the following are types of advance directives except ...

A. Living will

B. Durable power of attorney

C. Informed consent

D. DNR orders

24. Which of the following describes a nursing intervention?

A. A treatment order written by the physician and implemented by the nurse

B. It is used to meet specific client goals

C. Dependent nursing interventions require an order from an RN

D. Independent nursing interventions are created by an LPN

25. You are counseling a group of pregnant clients on the process of labor. Which of the following is not a sign of labor?

A. Show

B. Drainage of liquor

C. Blood clots

D. Waist pain

26. Which of the following is a component of the active management of the third stage of labor?

A. Prompt repair of lacerations and episiotomies.

B. Administering uterotonics to increase contractions

C. Administering adequate analgesia

D. Encouraging the mother to breastfeed

27. In reducing the risk of VAP (Ventilator-Associated Pneumonia), which of the following is correct?

A. Use nasal intubations instead of oral intubations unless contraindicated

B. Daily oral care with chlorhexidine solution is not necessary for nasal intubation

C. Endotracheal tubes with a subglottic port can prevent micro-aspiration

D. Endotracheal tubes with a bevel end can prevent micro-aspiration

28. Which of the following is true concerning safety measures to reduce catheter-related bloodstream infections (CRBSI)?

A. The femoral vein is the most preferred route for CVAC

B. Change peripheral lines every 48 hours

C. Clean injection ports with an isotonic fluid before each use

D. Change administration sets and add-in devices daily

29. Safety measures to reduce hospital-acquired UTIs include all of the following except ...

A. Use sterile gloves during catheterization to maintain asepsis

B. Maintain unobstructed urine flow by hanging the urine bag above the level of the bladder

C. The urinary bag should never make contact with the floor

D. Change urinary catheters every 36 hours

30. Concerning environmental safety measures, which of the following is correct?

A. Pathogens like MRSA, VRE and *Clostridium difficile* are susceptible and do not survive for long in non-organic environments

B. The ICU should be situated close to the main wards

C. Adequate space between beds is about two to three meters

D. Isolation facilities should have both positive and negative pressure rooms

31. Concerning safety measures in burn centers, which of the following is correct?

A. Shrubs and flowers can be planted to release more oxygen

B. Human tetanus immunoglobulin is not given to clients with active immunization

C. Topical antibiotics should be applied directly to a burn site

D. Systemic intravenous antibiotics are indicated for a short time

32. Concerning infection control for transplant patients, which of the following is correct?

A. Patients should be kept in rooms with negative-pressure ventilation

B. The most important safety precaution is handwashing

C. The most important safety precaution is prophylactic antibiotics

D. Live-attenuated and toxoid vaccines are useful for boosting active immunity

33. A mother wants to know how to care for her newborn's umbilical cord. Which of the following statements is incorrect?

A. The cord will fall off in two to four weeks

B. Give sponge baths to keep the stump dry

C. Do not pull the cord off

D. Fold the baby's diaper below the navel to prevent irritation

34. All of the following are measures to reduce risk of congenital malformations except ...

A. Prompt treatment of sexually transmitted infections

B. Avoid all forms of radiation

C. Commence prophylactic folic acid supplementation from 16 weeks of gestation

D. Avoid drugs contraindicated in pregnancy

35. Concerning the safety guidelines to reduce biohazards amongst health workers, all of the following are correct except ...

A. Inform health workers of possible effects of exposure to infectious agents

B. Educate health workers on various protocols for infectious diseases

C. Educate health workers on the proper use of PPE

D. Health-care workers with weeping infections of the hand shouldn't be excluded from direct contact with patients, as long as they wear sterile gloves

36. A female client is advised to do a hormone profile evaluation for secondary infertility. Which of the following is true?

A. FSH, LH and progesterone are assayed on day 3

B. Progesterone and estradiol are assayed on day 21

C. A high FSH indicates ovulation

D. Luteinizing hormone is released from the pituitary and ovaries

37. A child with acute nephritic syndrome will benefit from all of the following except ...

A. Strict fluid input/output monitoring

B. Restricted protein intake

C. Restricted salt intake

D. Bladder irrigation

38. All of the following are likely features of Potter's syndrome except ...

A. Hypoplastic lungs

B. Hydronephrosis

C. Oligohydramnios

D. Polyhydramnios

39. Which of the following clients is least at risk of having a urinary tract infection?

A. A two-week-old male with a posterior urethral valve

B. A female client with candidiasis

C. A quadriplegic patient with a neurogenic bladder

D. An elderly patient with urinary incontinence

40. Which of the following clinical parameters is used to assess kidney function?

A. Urine volume

B. Urine frequency

C. Urine color

D. Urine smell

41. All of the following are examples of renal causes of kidney injury except ...

A. Posterior urethral valve

B. Polycystic kidney disease

C. Nephritic syndrome

D. Nephrolithiasis

42. Concerning chronic kidney disease, which of the following management principles is incorrect?

A. Aspirin is given for chronic groin pain

B. Blood pressure is tightly controlled

C. Dialysis may be an option

D. Restricting sodium consumption may be beneficial

43. All of the following are causes of hematuria except ...

A. Sickle cell crisis

B. Acute nephritic syndrome

C. Porphyria

D. Pyelonephritis

44. A two-year-old male presents to the children's emergency ward with painful urination, high-grade fever, vomiting and abdominal pain. Which of the following treatment plans should be prioritized?

A. Provide pain relief

B. Commence empirical antibiotics

C. Control temperature

D. Monitor fluid input/output

45. All of the following are features of right-sided heart failure except ...

A. Pedal edema

B. Hepatomegaly

C. Ascites

D. Orthopnea

46. A client with left-sided heart failure is likely to have all of the following symptoms except ...

A. Orthopnea

B. Paroxysmal nocturnal tachypnea

C. Pedal edema

D. Cyanosis

47. A hypertensive client presents to the emergency room with chest pain, breathlessness and worsening cyanosis. Management principles for this patient may include all of the following except ...

A. Use of supplemental oxygen

B. Prompt cardiac compressions

C. Use of intravenous Lasix

D. Use of fibrinolytics

48. Concerning hypercalcemia, which of the following is true?

A. Serum calcium is greater than 2 mmol/L

B. Tetanic seizure is a complication

C. Hypothyroidism is a likely cause

D. It can be treated with calcitonin

49. All of the following are effects of hyperkalemia except ...

A. Arrhythmia

B. Numbness

C. Muscle weakness

D. Tetany

50. An obese patient has been admitted for post-op care. Early management should include which of the following?

A. Early ambulation

B. Elevating the foot of the bed

C. Daily weighing

D. Daily turning

51. All of the following are examples of cyanotic congenital heart diseases except ...

A. Tetralogy of Fallot

B. Tricuspid atresia

C. Ventricular septal defect

D. Transposition of the great arteries

52. In pediatric cardiopulmonary resuscitation, the ratio of cardiac massage to ventilation is?

A. 3:1

B. 2:1

C. 1:1

D. 2:2

53. A five-year-old child having Tet spells finds some relief by squatting. Which of the following statements correctly explains the reason?

A. Squatting increases pulmonary vascular resistance and pulmonary blood flow

B. Squatting decreases pressure on the left side of the heart

C. Squatting temporarily reverses the right-to-left shunt

D. Squatting increases pressure on the right side of the heart

54. Which of the following clients will benefit from a urinary catheter?

A. A 60-year-old client with Parkinson's disease and urinary incontinence

B. A 55-year-old male client with pedal edema caused by right-sided heart failure

C. A 23-year-old male client with a urethral stricture and acute urinary retention

D. A 50-year-old male client with chronic leg ulcers

55. Which of the following clients will benefit from a feeding tube?

A. A chemotherapy client with nausea and loss of appetite

B. An immunosuppressed client with oral candidiasis

C. A two-month-old female with breathlessness caused by acute heart failure

D. A road traffic accident client with a mild head injury

56. A 20-year-old woman presents to the neuropsychiatry clinic. Her BMI at presentation is 18 kg/m^2. Which of the following is correct?

A. This client is overweight

B. This client is underweight

C. This client is cachectic

D. This client is malnourished

57. A two-year-old child with a respiratory rate of 60 cpm has ...

A. A fast respiratory rate

B. A slow respiratory rate

C. A normal respiratory rate

D. Bronchial breath sounds

58. A two-month-old infant with a heart rate of 100 bpm has ...

A. A fast heart rate

B. A slow heart rate

C. A normal heart rate

D. A third heart sound

59. All of the following clients are at risk for aspiration except ...

A. A client with epileptic fits

B. A client with dysphagia

C. A pediatric client with a cleft lip

D. A client with aphasia

60. A client with constipation is at risk for all of the following except ...

A. Fecal impaction

B. Anal fissures

C. Fecal incontinence

D. Mallory–Weiss syndrome

61. A client with diabetes mellitus has an HbA1c of 12%. Which of the following is correct?

A. The client has an optimal glycemic control

B. The client is at risk for diabetic ketoacidosis

C. The client should be counseled on hypoglycemic emergencies

D. The client has impaired glucose tolerance

62. A gravid patient at 38 weeks presents to the emergency room with vaginal bleeding. She hasn't been compliant with her prenatal care. All of the following immediate actions are important except ...

A. A vaginal examination to assess the cause of bleeding

B. Resuscitation with fluids

C. Fetal heart monitoring

D. Requesting blood from the blood bank

63. A 45-year-old client with intestinal adhesions is suffering from severe vomiting and abdominal pain. This patient is increasingly lethargic. The client's arterial blood gases are as follows:

pH – 7.6

PaO2 – 86 mmHg

PaCO2 – 40 mmHg

HCO3 – 35 mmol/L

This client has ...

A. Metabolic alkalosis

B. Metabolic acidosis

C. Respiratory alkalosis

D. Respiratory acidosis

64. A known asthmatic client presents to the emergency room with chest tightness, wheezing, coughing and difficulty breathing. The client is confused and feels drowsy. The client's arterial blood gases are as follows:

pH – 7.35

PaCO2 – 72 mmHg

HCO3 – 35 mmol/L

This client has ...

A. Respiratory alkalosis

B. Metabolic acidosis

C. Respiratory acidosis

D. Metabolic alkalosis

65. Which of the following is not a likely cause of anaphylaxis?

A. Bee stings

B. Gluten

C. Oral Ibuprofen

D. Tuberculin bacilli

66. Concerning the principles of pain management, which of the following guidelines should be prioritized above others?

A. Acknowledge the client's perception of pain

B. Evaluate the efficacy and side effects of each pain medication

C. Involve caregivers in the implementation of pain management methods

D. Evaluate the client's risk of opioid dependence

67. A preeclamptic client is on magnesium sulfate therapy. Which of the following is a feature of magnesium sulfate toxicity?

A. Brisk, deep tendon reflexes

B. A respiratory rate of 16 cycles per minute

C. A urine output of 15 ml/hr

D. A blood pressure of 160/90 mmHg

68. Which of the following is not a routine drug for prenatal care?

A. Fersolate

B. Folic acid

C. Vitamin C

D. Vitamin A

69. Concerning a hypertensive client on an ACE inhibitor, which of the following statements is correct?

A. Needs routine investigation of serum sodium

B. May complain of a cough

C. May be pregnant

D. May require potassium supplements

70. Which of the following blood products is ideal for a two-year-old hemophiliac in hemorrhagic shock?

A. Platelet concentrate

B. Red blood cells

C. Fresh frozen plasma

D. Fresh whole blood

71. Why are corticosteroids not readily used with children?

A. They increase a child's susceptibility to fungal infections

B. They increase blood pressure

C. They reduce bone growth and density

D. They increase serum glucose levels

72. Concerning acetylsalicylic acid, which of the following is correct?

A. It can be taken on an empty stomach

B. It can be taken with antacids

C. It can cause tinnitus

D. It can be used as an antihypertensive

73. Which of the following is true concerning a chemical name?

A. It's also known as the generic name

B. It's also known as the scientific name

C. It's also known as the non-proprietary name

D. It's usually shortened to a prefix

74. A doctor writes a prescription order for tabs rosuvastatin 20 mg nocte. Rosuvastatin is an example of which of the following drug names?

A. Trade name

B. Generic name

C. Brand name

D. Chemical name

75. A doctor writes a prescription order for tabs Viagra 50 mg daily. Which of the following is correct concerning Viagra?

A. It is a proprietary name

B. The trade name is sildenafil

C. The chemical name is sildenafil

D. It can be used to treat hypotension

76. Drug A is prescribed to increase the action of Drug B. This drug action is called ...

A. Agonism

B. Synergism

C. Potentiation

D. Cataclysm

77. Which of the following drug actions is not an example of synergism?

A. A combination of penicillin and gentamycin

B. A combination of penicillin and probenecid

C. A combination of aspirin and caffeine

D. A combination of allopurinol and methotrexate

78. First-line anti-Koch's do not include ...

A. Pyrazinamide

B. Ethambutol

C. Streptomycin

D. Rifampicin

79. A client on anti-Koch's complains of blurry vision and objects appearing washed out. Which of the following drugs is implicated?

A. Rifampicin

B. Ethambutol

C. Isoniazid

D. Pyrazinamide

80. Two brothers, aged 11 months and 5 years, present to the dermatology clinic. Their mother gives a history of itchy rashes in the groin, fingers and toes. A diagnosis of scabies is made. The 11-month-old male will benefit from any of these drugs except ...

A. Benzyl Benzoate

B. Permethrin

C. Lindane

D. Loratadine

81. A two-week-old neonate with VSD will benefit from any of the following drugs except ...

A. Ibuprofen

B. Indomethacin

C. Caffeine

D. Acetaminophen

82. All of the following can give relief to a client with constipation except ...

A. Dulcolax

B. Milk of magnesia

C. Lomotil

D. Bisacodyl

83. Which of the following clients is in need of a white cane?

A. A client with Parkinson's disease

B. A client with osteoarthritis of the hip

C. A client with macular degeneration in both eyes

D. A client with a complete cervical spine transection

84. You are to counsel a client on proper care for a colostomy. Which of the following guidelines is incorrect?

A. Empty a colostomy pouch only when it is completely full

B. Use skin-barrier products to prevent dermatitis

C. Eat a variety of healthy foods for adequate nutrition

D. Drink enough water to stay hydrated

85. Which of these colostomy complications is correctly matched to its explanation?

A. Stenosis – occurs when the stoma sinks below the skin level

B. Prolapse – a part of the bowel pushes out of the stoma

C. Hernia – occurs when the stoma lumen narrows

D. Retraction – occurs when a part of the bowel pushes out of the area around the stoma

86. You need to collect a urine sample from a two-year-old male. Which of the following methods is suitable?

A. Use a three-way urethral catheter

B. Use a two-way urethral catheter

C. Do a clean catch

D. Suction the urine from the child's diaper

87. All of the following interventions are beneficial in reducing secretions in a client with a tracheostomy except ...

A. Encouraging the client to cough out secretions

B. Suctioning every two hours

C. Providing warm and humidified air

D. Assessing changes in heart rate, respiratory rate and temperature

88. All of the following interventions are beneficial in controlling the temperature of a child with acute rheumatic fever except ...

A. Giving NSAIDs to reduce the temperature

B. Giving a tepid sponge bath

C. Removing excess clothing

D. Restricting fluid intake to prevent congestive cardiac failure

89. All of the following are nursing interventions to increase calorie intake in a client with chronic bronchitis except ...

A. Frequent care of the oral cavity

B. Encouraging the client to eat small, frequent meals

C. Increasing fluid intake during meals

D. Serving food hot to prevent spasms

90. A client can't stop using marijuana because he says nothing else makes him feel happy and powerful. Your client has what type of dependency?

A. Physical

B. Psychological

C. Sociological

D. Mental

91. You are caring for a suicidal client. Which of the following responses should be prioritized?

A. Discuss the moral implications of suicide with your client

B. Keep your client in a bare and empty room

C. Assess the possible risk factors for your client

D. Examine your feelings and beliefs about suicide

92. Which of the following care plans should be prioritized for a client with dementia?

A. Provide good nutrition

B. Improve water intake

C. Provide a safe environment with good security

D. Commence physiotherapy

93. A female client presents to the emergency unit. Her significant other gives a history of sudden onset of loss of personal ideation, visual hallucinations and confused speech. Your diagnosis is most likely delirium because, unlike dementia, delirium has which of the following distinguishing characteristics?

A. Prevalence in females

B. Sudden onset

C. Visual hallucinations

D. Confused speech

94. A female client is admitted for bulimia nervosa. Which of the following is the characteristic feature of bulimia?

A. Episodic binge eating and induced vomiting

B. Low self-esteem

C. Body dysmorphia

D. Low body mass

95. Which of the following characteristics distinguishes malingering from a somatoform disorder?

A. Involuntary

B. Voluntary

C. Organic

D. Physiological

96. Which of the following activities has a low risk of triggering anorexia?

A. Ballet

B. Modeling

C. Boxing

D. Tennis

97. During an abdominal examination, a healthy liver is expected to produce which of the following sounds on percussion?

A. Tympanic

B. Dull

C. Stony dull

D. Resonant

98. In a cardiac examination of a hypertensive client, you observe that the client's apex beat was located at the seventh LICS, MCL. This client most likely has which of the following?

A. An impending cardiac tamponade

B. A pneumothorax

C. A ventricular dilatation

D. A pleural effusion

99. Which of the following cranial nerve examinations is incorrect?

A. Pupillary reflex – Cranial nerve III

B. Hearing – Cranial nerve VII

C. Soap – Cranial nerve I

D. Corneal reflex – Cranial nerve III

100. Finger clubbing is least likely in which of the following clients?

A. A two-year-old male with a tetralogy of Fallot

B. A 74-year-old man with a decompensated liver disease

C. A 25-year-old male with inflammatory bowel disease

D. A premature two-week-old male with a PDA

Answers to Test 1

1. (D) Personal beliefs.

A scholarly journal is an academic work that gives researchers an opportunity to contribute to knowledge. Scholarly journals provide verifiable evidence for their claims.

2. (C) Experimental research.

Qualitative research uses both unstructured and semi-structured methods to obtain non-numerical data. The aim of qualitative research is to explore phenomena. This involves describing variations and relationships between data, describing individual experiences and describing group norms. The main types of qualitative research include the phenomenological model, the ethnographic model, the grounded theory model, the case study model, the narrative model and the historical model.

3. (B) Brand of glucometer.

This variable can be changed in this experiment. It is the variable you can control. It is also called a controlled variable.

4. (A) Sensitivities of glucometers.

This variable is the condition that can be measured in this experiment. It is also called the responding variable.

5. (B) Hepatic drug clearance.

Reduced hepatic function in the elderly is an important factor to consider in drug pharmacodynamics because the elderly have reduced hepatic clearance. Therefore, the accumulation of drugs and adverse effects are likely risks.

6. (D) Narrow therapeutic index.

Polypharmacy is the use of multiple drugs by a patient. It is a common occurrence in the elderly and can increase the risks of adverse drug reactions, non-compliance and drug-drug interaction. It, however, has no effect on the therapeutic index of a drug.

7. (C) A diastolic murmur is a low-frequency sound.

Option A is incorrect because high-frequency sounds are assessed with the diaphragm of the stethoscope. Option B is incorrect because low-pitched sounds are assessed with the bell of the stethoscope. Option D is incorrect because the apex beat is a high-frequency sound.

8. (B) Clotting profile.

A clotting profile isn't necessary prior to a red blood cell transfusion. A hematocrit is used to assess the hemoglobin level; serology is used to screen the client for blood diseases like HIV, hepatitis and syphilis; and blood grouping and cross-matching is needed to assess the recipient's blood group to reduce the risk of blood transfusion reactions.

9. (C) Air is a radiopaque substance.

Air is a radiolucent substance that appears dark on the film. It doesn't absorb as many x-rays as radiopaque substances.

10. (A) They are interdependent nursing interventions implemented with other health-care professionals.

Collaborative nursing interventions are done in partnership with other health-care professionals. The aim of this intervention is to provide holistic and patient-centered nursing care to patients. These interventions aren't necessarily supervised by a medical doctor or a leader on a nursing team.

11. (B) It is also known as nosocomial pneumonia.

Hospital-acquired pneumonia is also known as nosocomial pneumonia. Option A is incorrect because symptoms appear more than 48 hours after admission in patients with no evidence of infection prior to admission. Option C is incorrect because the most common cause is a bacterial infection like *Staph aureus*. Option D is incorrect because the use of systemic steroids is a risk factor that increases susceptibility to HAP.

12. (D) A single nurse is the primary caregiver of the client.

In a primary nursing care model, a single nurse is responsible for a patient. Option A is incorrect because it is a characteristic of team-based nursing. Option B is incorrect because it is a feature for functional nursing. Option C is incorrect because it is a feature of the floating nursing model.

13. (B) The client's geographic location.

In modular nursing, nurses are allocated based on the client's geographic location in the hospital.

14. (C) African American.

Keloids are prevalent amongst sub-Saharan Africans, African Americans and Asians.

15. (A) Chinese American.

A Chinese American person is most likely to avoid direct eye contact as a show of respect for personal space.

16. (C) Paraphrasing.

In paraphrasing, the listener attempts to interpret and summarize the emotional content of the speaker's words. The aim of this technique is to let the speaker know that his/her intent is understood. Option A is incorrect because in offering self, the nurse shows that she is available for communication. Option B is incorrect because probing is a non-therapeutic communication technique that makes use of close-ended questions to lead a client on and get more information that is then used to make an evaluation. Option D is incorrect because giving recognition is a therapeutic communication technique that makes use of observation skills to acknowledge a client's actions without giving compliments.

17. (C) Making observation.

In this technique, the listener notices changes in the speaker's appearance and demeanor. The purpose of this technique is to interpret nonverbal communication from the speaker and encourage the speaker to talk further. This technique is also used to discover new symptoms.

18. (C) Fidelity is synonymous with faithfulness.

Option A is incorrect because justice is synonymous with fairness. Option B is incorrect because nonmaleficence means doing no intentional and unintentional harm to the client. Option D is incorrect because accountability means holding oneself accountable for one's actions.

19. (D) The World Nurses Association.

The World Nurses Association is a fictional regulatory body.

20. (A) Routine handwashing.

Primary prevention methods eliminate the risks of diseases. Handwashing is a preventive measure that reduces the risk of transmission of infectious diseases that are spread through aerosols, droplet nuclei, direct contact and feco-oral routes. Options B and D are secondary prevention methods. Option C is a tertiary prevention method.

21. (B) Hypoactive bowel sounds can indicate an intestinal obstruction.

In intestinal obstruction, bowel sounds are increased in frequency and are high-pitched. Disease conditions where hypoactive bowel sounds are heard include but are not limited to paralytic ileus and peritonitis.

22. (B) Diabetes mellitus.

In diabetes mellitus, there are excess triglycerides and glucose in the blood. An excess of these nutrients impairs wound healing. Option A is incorrect because cobalamin deficiency causes megaloblastic anemia. Option C is incorrect because the client has a normal BMI. Option D is incorrect because the client has normal serum sodium.

23. (C) Help mothers initiate breastfeeding within 24 hours of birth.

Breastfeeding is initiated in the first hour of birth. Benefits of prompt breastfeeding include but are not limited to bonding between the mother and child; secretion of prolactin, which can help the uterus to contract; secretion of colostrum to protect the infant from certain infectious diseases and prevention of neonatal hypoglycemia.

24. (C) The baby's nose should be opposite the mother's areola.

For proper attachment during breastfeeding, the baby's nose should be opposite the mother's nipple and not the areola. This position helps the baby have the entire nipple and areola in its mouth. Proper attachment ensures adequate feeding for the baby, sufficient drainage of the breast, continuous milk supply and less nipple pain.

25. (A) IgA.

Colostrum is the milk produced as soon as lactation commences. Although it is rich in other antibodies, colostrum has a significant amount of secretory IgA, which gives the newborn passive immunity to infectious diseases of the gastrointestinal and respiratory system.

26. (C) Cough into your hands and wash them off immediately if a tissue isn't available.

It is not safe to cough into your hands because there is an increased risk of spreading infectious droplets either through direct contact (like handshakes) or indirect contact (like touching doorknobs and handrails). Clients are counseled to cough into the inner part of their elbow instead of into their hands.

27. (B) Tofu and mixed vegetable salad with quinoa.

Clients with gluten intolerance have allergic reactions to gluten that is contained in cereal grains like wheat, spelt and rye. Option A is incorrect because it has mixed grains, which could include gluten cereals. Option C is incorrect because it has spaghetti, which is made from wheat. Option D is incorrect because it has a wheat bagel.

28. (D) Kubler Ross' theory of grief.

Kubler Ross' stages of grief model is used to manage the terminally ill and their relatives. The stages of grief include denial, anger, bargaining, depression and acceptance. Option A is incorrect because Warden's theory is used for helping people who recently lost a loved one to accept and cope with loss. Option B is incorrect because Engel's theory of grief includes the stages of grief that occur weeks or months prior to the loss of a loved one.

29. (B) The child will benefit from a structured and controlled environment.

Children with ADHD are easily distracted, restless, forgetful and impulsive. This client will benefit from a structured and controlled environment. Option A is incorrect because children with autism prefer routines and inanimate objects. Option D is incorrect because children with conduct disorder have a history of stealing, lying and truancy.

30. (A) Behavioral therapy.

Behavioral therapy is used to treat mild depression and somatoform disorders. It involves the identification of negative thoughts and the replacement of these negative thoughts with positive ones. Option B is incorrect because aversive conditioning is used to treat paraphilias or addiction. Option C is incorrect because flooding and implosion are used to treat phobias.

31. (B) Regression.

In regression, the client attempts to cope with stress by retreating to an earlier developmental stage.

32. (B) Projection.

Clients with paranoid disorders usually project their distrust and paranoia on others. For example, a client with paranoid disorder may believe that people hate him and are out to get him.

33. (C) The cognitive model.

The cognitive model focuses on improving the existing abilities of a client with a disability. Option A is incorrect because the biomedical model is focused on treating and managing disabilities. Option B is incorrect because the social model focuses on the attitudes and systemic biases that make it hard for clients with disabilities to function in society. Option D is incorrect because there is no pathological model of disability.

34. (C) Pica.

Pica is a craving for substances without nutritive value. Although people attribute pica to one of the symptoms of pregnancy, a health worker should investigate the cause even if the client is pregnant. Most times, the craving can come from a nutrient deficiency. Pica is a common feature of iron deficiency. Clients can crave substances like ice, clay, cigarette ash, sand, dust and buttons. Complications of pica include heavy-metal poisoning, choking, parasitic infections and intestinal obstruction.

35. (A) Substance abuse.

A client has a substance abuse disorder when he/she continues to take a prescription drug even when there is no more indication for using the drug. Substance abuse can lead to addiction and physical and psychological dependence.

36. (B) An air bed.

A bedridden patient is at risk of developing pressure ulcers at pressure points such as the sacrum, coccyx, hip bones, heels and elbows. Beds filled with air/water support the client's weight with little friction between the client's body and the bed surface.

37. (B) Diapers.

Diapers are convenient and suitable for this client. Option A is incorrect because a urethral catheter increases the risk of urinary tract infections and isn't suitable for long-term use. Option C is incorrect because a bedpan is not useful for a client with incontinence. Option D is incorrect because a cystostomy is a surgical procedure done for clients with bladder outlet obstructions caused by urethral strictures.

38. (C) Engage the client in weight-bearing exercises.

Due to immobility, there is increased calcium resorption from the bones and into the blood. This action is triggered by the osteolytic action of osteoclasts in the bone matrix. Weight-bearing exercises stimulate the formation of osteoblasts and positive bone remodeling.

39. (C) A pad and a pen.

Aphasia is an inability to form comprehensible language due to damage to the speech area of the cerebral cortex. This client is literate and will benefit from using a pad and a pen to communicate. Option A is incorrect because, although a bell can be used by the client to raise an alarm, it is not useful for communication. Option B is incorrect because a hearing aid is not indicated since the client isn't deaf.

40. (D) Slippers.

Clients with Parkinson's are at great risk of sustaining injuries from falls. It is advisable that they avoid materials with little traction, such as traditional slippers, rugs, and socks that don't have non-slip soles.

41. (D) Place the patient in the Sims position.

The Sims position is also called the lateral recumbent position. The patient lies on his/her left side, with the left hip and lower limb kept straight. The right hip and right knee are bent. This position is used for rectal examinations and enemas. In the given scenario, the client should be placed in the High Fowler's position to prevent aspiration of gastric contents into the respiratory airway.

42. (A) Foods rich in plant fiber.

Fiber increases the enterohepatic circulation and excretion of cholesterol in the feces. Although unsaturated fat is not as harmful as saturated fat and cholesterol, foods high in fat can cause obesity and worsen heart disease.

43. (A) 14–17 hours.

Neonates sleep for a total of 14–17 hours a day. They typically sleep for 8–9 hours at night, waking up in between to feed.

44. (B) 2.5 ml.

If 1 ml = 20 mg

and X ml = 50 mg,

X = 50 mg ÷ 20 mg

X = 2.5 ml.

45. (A) 2.5 tablets.

If 1 tablet = 100 mg

and X tablets = 250 mg,

X = 250 mg ÷ 100 mg

X = 2.5 tablets.

46. (C) Diarrhea.

Diarrhea is not a likely complication because TPN bypasses the alimentary canal. Instead, macro- and micronutrients are shunted directly into the circulation. Other risks of TPN include hyperglycemia, fatty liver, liver failure, dehydration, refeeding syndrome, hunger pangs, electrolyte imbalance and micronutrient deficiencies. Also, air embolisms and sepsis are likely complications, as seen in other parenteral therapies.

47. (A) Universal red blood cell donor.

The O negative blood group has neither A nor B antigens in the red blood cells. It also doesn't have D antigens. The lack of these antigens makes O negative blood universally acceptable for red blood cell transfusions. The AB negative blood group is the universal plasma cell donor because, although it has both A and B antigens in the red blood cells, it has no A and B antibodies in the plasma.

48. (D) The donor has only A and B antibodies.

The B blood group has B antigens in the red blood cells and A antibodies in the plasma. This recipient doesn't have the rhesus D antigen, so he is RHd negative.

The O blood group has neither A nor B antigens in the red blood cells. It does, however, have the A and B antibodies in the plasma. This donor doesn't have the rhesus D antigen, so he is RHd negative.

49. (A) The lesser trochanter.

IM medications are administered in the ventrogluteal aspect of the buttocks. To do this, the administration site is identified by placing the heel of the hand on the greater trochanter. The thumb is pointed toward the belly button and the index finger extended to the anterior superior iliac spine. The middle finger is pointed towards the iliac crest. Medications are given in the V groove formed between the index and middle fingers.

50. (C) Penicillin.

The therapeutic window is used in pharmacology to measure the range of drug doses that give a therapeutic response without causing any significant adverse effect in patients. Therapeutic windows are used to measure the therapeutic index/therapeutic ratio, a quantitative measurement of the relative safety of a drug. Drugs with low therapeutic indexes have an unfavorable safety profile. Examples include lithium, digoxin and acetaminophen. On the other end, penicillin has a wide therapeutic window and a high therapeutic index.

51. (C) ESR.

An erythrocyte sedimentation rate is used to measure the rate at which red blood cells settle at the bottom of a test tube. Normal red blood cells settle slowly. A faster-than-normal sedimentation rate indicates inflammation. ESR is used to diagnose both acute and chronic inflammatory processes and monitor a client's response to antibiotics. However, it has no influence on the pharmacokinetics of anesthetic drugs.

52. (D) PCV.

Packed cell volume is a measure of the percentage of hemoglobin volume in the blood. It is used to diagnose anemia and polycythemia but not bleeding disorders. The components of a clotting profile include international normalized ratio (INR), prothrombin time (PT) and partial thromboplastin time (PTT).

Warfarin is an anticoagulant used for clients in thrombotic/embolic states. Bleeding is a common side effect of warfarin. To reduce the incidence of bleeding, the clotting profile of the client is routinely monitored.

53. (D) Size 26G.

This cannula is purple. It has a length of 19 mm, an external diameter of 0.6 mm and a flow rate of 13 ml/min. This cannula is preferable for neonates because their veins are fragile and tiny, with small lumens. Because of this, a neonate's veins are susceptible to trauma. Size 16G, 18G and 20G cannulae are longer, wider and not suitable for pediatric use.

54. (C) It is compatible with an AB recipient.

The A blood group type has A antigens in the red blood cells and B antibodies in the plasma. This makes it incompatible with the AB blood group type. Since the AB blood group has both A and B antigens in red blood cells, it is an incompatible donor for the B blood group but is a compatible recipient.

55. (D) Dextrose water.

Emergency resuscitation fluids include colloids and crystalloids like Hartmann's solution and normal saline. Colloids contain proteins with large molecular weights. These molecules exert a high oncotic pressure and thus keep fluids in the intravascular compartment. They include human albumin, dextran and Haemaccel.

0.9% normal saline and Hartmann's solution both spread through the intravascular and interstitial spaces, thus making them useful as both resuscitation and maintenance fluids. However, dextrose water infusions are only used as maintenance fluids because they don't equilibrate across the interstitial and intravascular spaces.

56. (B) It is associated with vesicant drugs.

Extravasation occurs when an intravenous catheter is dislodged and a vesicant drug is infused into the tissue. Clinical features of extravasation include swelling, redness, stinging and local necrosis. Treatment modalities include the application of cold compresses, use of an antidote and debridement in cases of tissue necrosis.

57. (A) It is usually associated with alkaline solutions.

Phlebitis is an inflammation of a peripheral vein. It is usually caused by alkaline and acidic solutions, and also solutions with high osmolarity. Option B is incorrect because the treatment modalities include the application of warm and moist compresses. Option D is incorrect because chemotherapy drugs are vesicants that can cause extravasation.

58. (B) 0.9% normal saline is a likely cause.

Infiltration occurs when a non-vesicant drug is infused into the surrounding tissue. Option A is incorrect because 50% dextrose water has high osmolarity and can cause phlebitis. Options C and D are incorrect because IV paclitaxel and IV vancomycin are vesicant drugs that can cause extravasation.

59. (B) Hepatic encephalopathy.

This client is most likely in decompensated liver failure and is at risk of developing hepatic encephalopathy from impaired ammonia excretion. To reduce the risk of ammonia accumulation, interventions like hydration, restriction of protein and improvement of bowel motility are employed.

60. (B) She is at risk of developing eclamptic fits.

This client has preeclampsia, a hypertensive disease of pregnancy characterized by hypertension and proteinuria. She is at risk of developing eclamptic fits, an obstetric emergency that is characterized by neurological symptoms, blood coagulopathies and multiorgan failure.

61. (C) Provide supplemental oxygen.

This client is hypoxic and is in urgent need of oxygen supplementation. His cardiovascular status is fairly stable; therefore, a vasoconstrictor and resuscitation with intravenous fluids aren't indicated for acute management.

62. (B) Hydrate the client with normal saline.

This client has diabetic ketoacidosis and is severely dehydrated. He is also at risk of going into hypovolemic shock. Immediate care includes rehydration with about 6–8 L of normal saline. Other interventions include an assessment of the client's dehydration status, urine output and level of consciousness. Intravenous insulin is given, not subcutaneous insulin.

63. (C) The landmarks for measuring this client's OFC are the glabella and the occiput.

Option A is incorrect because macrocephaly is an OFC that is greater than the 98th percentile. Option D is incorrect because microcephaly is an OFC that is less than the third percentile. The landmarks for measuring the OFC include the occiput, the glabella or just above the supraorbital ridge.

64. (A) Obesity is a weight that is greater than or equal to the 95th percentile.

Option B is incorrect because underweight is a BMI that is below the fifth percentile. Options C and D are incorrect because BMI is not a direct measurement of body fat and is measured in kilograms per square meter.

65. (D) Transfuse with red blood cells.

This client is severely anemic and is therefore unfit for chemotherapy. The client should be transfused with at least three units of packed cells or until he is hemodynamically stable. Bone marrow suppression is a common complication of chemotherapy. Option B is incorrect because the client's white blood cell count is normal and he shows no signs of infection. Option C is incorrect because the client's platelet count is normal.

66. (B) Hemodialysis.

This client has azotemia and is at risk of developing arrhythmia and uremic encephalopathy. He also meets the clinical indication for hemodialysis. Option A is incorrect because dextrose insulin infusion is used for mild cases of hyperkalemia. Option C is incorrect because there is no clinical information that shows that this client has a fluid overload. Option D is incorrect because a potassium-sparing antihypertensive is not an emergency treatment for this client's azotemia.

67. (B) Calcium 3.5 mEq/L.

This client has hypocalcemia. The normal range of serum calcium is 4.3–5.2 mEq/L. The features of hypocalcemia include numbness, muscle spasm, confusion, seizures and cardiac arrest. The possible causes of hypocalcemia include hypoparathyroidism, vitamin D deficiency, kidney failure, calcium channel blockers and pancreatitis.

68. (B) Cholesterol 6.5 mmol/L.

This client has hypercholesterolemia. The desirable range for serum cholesterol values is less than 5.2 mmol/L. This client is at risk for atherosclerosis and cardiovascular diseases such as hypertension, stroke, myocardial infarction and peripheral artery disease.

69. (A) Compartment syndrome.

This client is likely to have compartment syndrome, a painful condition caused by the increasing pressure of tissues in anatomical compartments. It is a common complication seen in patients wearing a cast. Compartment syndrome is an orthopedic emergency that requires quick intervention and relief of the rising pressure. Features of compartment syndrome include the 5 Ps: pain, pallor, paresthesia, pulselessness and paralysis.

70. (B) A client with a GCS of 3.

This client has a severe head injury with loss of motor, sensory and cognitive function. He is at risk of developing pressure ulcers on the weight-bearing areas like the hips, elbows and ankles. The nursing care interventions required to reduce the risk of pressure ulcers include two-hourly turning, regular skin assessments, and preventing moisture, shearing and friction.

71. (D) A 40-year-old female with a goiter.

Causes of hypocalcemia include vitamin D insufficiency, hypoparathyroidism, calcium deficiency, end-stage renal disease and total or partial thyroidectomies. A disease of the parathyroid glands can cause hypothyroidism. A goiter is a disease of the thyroid glands and not the parathyroid glands.

72. (C) Iron therapy.

Sickle cell anemia is an autosomal recessive disorder of the red blood cells. This disorder causes the production and release of red blood cells that are sickled and sticky. These red blood cells are fragile and lyse easily. Iron therapy isn't useful to a client with sickle cell anemia because the excess hemolysis of red blood cells releases iron into the bloodstream. A sickle cell client is already at risk for iron overload. Therefore, iron therapy is contraindicated. Treatment options for sickle cell anemia include improvement of blood circulation, prevention of crises and management of complications.

73. (B) Anemia.

Cyanosis occurs when the deoxygenated hemoglobin level is above 5 g/dL. Because of this, patients with anemia do not develop cyanosis until the oxygen saturation falls below normal hemoglobin levels. Patients with anemia need lower oxygen saturation of about 50% before cyanosis becomes clinically apparent.

74. (B) A client who has received a shot of homologous human globulin.

Active immunity occurs when antibodies are produced as a response to the presence of an antigen. These antigens can be natural, as in the case of natural active immunity to chicken pox, or artificial, as in the cases of live-attenuated vaccines. Passive immunity occurs when an individual receives antibodies either naturally from breast milk or artificially via the administration of human globulins and antitoxins.

75. (C) There is decreased insulin sensitivity.

Although type 2 diabetes mellitus is prevalent in adults, it is neither a disease of adulthood nor of childhood. Unlike type 1 diabetes mellitus, type 2 is caused by a decreased sensitivity to insulin. As a result, the pancreas secretes higher amounts of insulin until the secreting glands burn out and are unable to secrete further insulin. Insulin is not the first treatment of choice. Lifestyle changes like dietary changes and exercise are first employed. If sugar is uncontrolled, oral hypoglycemic agents are added. Insulin is the last line of drug options.

76. (C) Hyperpigmentation.

Hyperpigmentation is a feature of Addison's disease, an endocrine disorder of insufficient cortisol production. Addison's can be caused by chronic diseases like tuberculosis and pituitary disorders, where little adrenocorticotropic hormone (ACTH) is released. Cushing's disease is an endocrine disorder of excess cortisol production. The symptoms of Cushing's disease include truncal obesity, striae, moon facies, stunting, hypertension, easy bruising, diabetes mellitus, hyperglycemia and cataracts.

77. (D) Enuresis.

Undiagnosed type 1 diabetics are most likely to present to the clinic with enuresis (bedwetting). Sudden onset of bedwetting in older children is likely to alert parents, who may miss other symptoms. Although diabetic ketoacidosis is the usual presentation, parents typically present children with this to the emergency room, and not the endocrinology clinic.

78. (B) Calcium.

Hypoparathyroidism is a likely complication of a total thyroidectomy. Because the parathyroid glands have a close relation to the thyroid, they can be injured, removed or have their blood supply impaired. Since parathyroid hormones control the metabolism of calcium, hypocalcemia is a likely complication of a total thyroidectomy.

79. (A) Use a foot antiperspirant daily.

This client has early signs of diabetic neuropathy. Such a patient is at risk of diabetic foot ulcers. A diabetic foot ulcer is a complication of uncontrolled diabetes mellitus. Impaired neurovascular function to the feet predisposes diabetics to ulcers, gangrene and foot deformities. The aim of foot care is to improve circulation and avoid injury and infections.

80. (A) Severe dehydration can cause hypovolemic shock.

Diabetic ketoacidosis is an example of metabolic acidosis. Ketosis, increased hydrogen ions and hyperglycemia all increase the blood's osmolarity. Because of this, a client with diabetic ketoacidosis is severely dehydrated.

Option B is incorrect because excess blood sugar does not trigger hemolysis. Options C and D are incorrect because although excess blood sugar triggers neuropathy and nephropathy, these conditions are chronic complications, not emergencies.

81. (A) Impaired glucose tolerance.

The normal range of fasting blood sugar is 3.5–5.5 mmol/L. Impaired glucose tolerance ranges from 5.5 mmol/L–6.5 mmol/L. Values greater than 6.5 mmol/L are diagnostic of diabetes mellitus. Impaired glucose tolerance is also called prediabetes. Such clients have a high risk of developing diabetes in the future.

82. (B) Dopamine.

Parkinson's disease is a neurodegenerative disease of the central nervous system. It is characterized by insufficient secretion of dopamine in the substantia nigra, located in the midbrain. Lewy bodies accumulate in the neurons of the substantia nigra, leading to cell death. The loss of these neurons reduces the amount of dopamine produced.

83. (C) Anisocoria.

Anisocoria is defined as a difference of 0.4 mm or more between the sizes of the pupils of the eyes. Ptosis is defined as a drooping of the eyelids. Miosis is defined as a constriction of the pupils, while mydriasis is defined as a dilatation of the pupils.

84. (D) It is part of the fight or flight response.

Miosis is a constriction of the pupils caused by stimulation and action of the parasympathetic nervous system. The flight or fight response is a function of the sympathetic nervous system. In the fight or flight response, mydriasis occurs, i.e., the pupils dilate to allow more light into the retina.

85. (A) Anterograde amnesia.

Anterograde amnesia is an inability to create new memories after the event that caused the amnesia. This causes a partial or complete inability to recall the recent past. However, long-term memories from before the event remain intact. In retrograde amnesia, memories prior to the event are lost, while new memories can still be made.

86. (B) It's caused by a block to the sympathetic pathway.

Horner's syndrome is a disorder of sympathetic origin. It occurs when a group of nerves known as the sympathetic trunk is damaged. The signs and symptoms occur on the same side, where the lesion on the sympathetic trunk is located. It is characterized by miosis, partial ptosis, anhidrosis and enophthalmos.

87. (C) Cyanosis.

Chronic liver disease is a progressive disease of the liver that leads to cirrhosis and fibrosis. Clinical signs/stigmata of this disease can be pathognomonic of either compensated or decompensated liver disease. These signs do not include cyanosis. Cyanosis is a clinical feature of impaired oxygenation in the red blood cells.

88. (C) A pediatric client with rotavirus infection.

Contact isolation is used for isolating clients with infections that are spread through contact. These include skin infections, gastrointestinal infections spread through the feco-oral route and from the hands to the mouth. Personal protection equipment like gloves and gowns is necessary.

Options A and D are prevented by airborne and droplet isolation. Option B is a sexually transmitted infection.

89. (C) A client with aspiration pneumonitis.

Aspiration pneumonitis is a lung inflammation caused by aspiration of substances that irritate and traumatize the respiratory airway. Since it is not caused by microbial infections, isolation protocols for infectious diseases are not necessary.

90. (C) It is a form of isolation that protects a client from the environment.

This form of isolation protects the client from contact, respiratory and droplet routes of infection. Reverse isolation is practiced in rooms with laminar airflow and strict handwashing hygiene. It is suitable for clients with severe immunosuppression. This client has severe immunosuppression due to leukopenia and is eligible for reverse isolation.

91. (B) Wash your hands.

Handwashing is the first safety measure in preventing and reducing the transmission of most communicable diseases. It prevents cross-contamination from the client to your hands and to the personal protective equipment. Handwashing is a universal precaution observed for all isolation protocols, whether respiratory, contact or droplet measures.

92. (C) Placing throw rugs in hallways.

Throw rugs increase the risks of this client falling, tripping or slipping. As such, throw rugs should be avoided or replaced with non-skid mats. Proper lighting improves visibility. Handrails and grab rails will improve stability and coordination when climbing the stairs or getting into bathtubs.

93. (C) They can be transferred through kissing.

Some sexually transmitted infections are transmitted through the saliva. Examples include the Herpes simplex virus and cytomegalovirus. Option A is incorrect because hormonal contraceptives protect against pregnancy, not infections. Option B is incorrect because the varicella-zoster virus is not a sexually transmitted infection. Option D is incorrect because bacterial vaginosis is not a sexually transmitted infection, although it increases the risk of its transmission.

94. (D) Bronze baby syndrome – keep phototherapy lights no more than 30.5 cm away from the neonate.

Bronze baby syndrome is a complication of phototherapy in neonates with conjugated hyperbilirubinemia. It is transient and disappears when phototherapy is discontinued.

95. (C) Visitors are to stay at least six feet away from the client's bed.

Visitors are to stay at least six feet away from the client who has just had a radiotherapy treatment. All the other options are correct.

96. (D) Confusion – give anxiolytics.

Confusion is a usual side effect of electroconvulsive therapy. Clients may experience confusion immediately after treatment. This can last from a few minutes to several hours. Clients are not given anxiolytics and are encouraged to take bed rest.

97. (D) Reduce the length of hospital admission.

Option A is incorrect because contact isolation measures are observed for MRSA. Option B is incorrect because steroids are not used for postoperative care since they are immunosuppressive. Option C is incorrect because there is currently no vaccine for MRSA.

98. (B) Immunization.

Immunization is the most effective method of reducing the incidence of bacterial and viral diseases of the respiratory and gastrointestinal tracts.

99. (D) Probiotics can prevent future occurrences.

Although probiotics are safe and beneficial in shortening the duration of diarrhea and reducing stool frequency in acute infective diarrhea, probiotics don't prevent the future occurrence of rotavirus-induced gastroenteritis.

100. (C) Despair.

Kubler Ross' five stages of grief are denial, anger, bargaining, depression and acceptance.

Answers to Test 2

1. (D) Human tissues.

The yellow container is for disposing of infected biodegradable materials like human tissues, cotton swabs, beddings and animal tissues. Option A is incorrect because cytotoxic drugs are disposed of in the black waste container. Option B is incorrect because infected plastics are disposed of in the red waste container. Option C is incorrect because used sharps are disposed of in the white waste container.

2. (D) White.

The white container is for disposing of infected and used sharps like surgical blades, lancets and syringes. The yellow container is for disposing of infectious non-plastic materials. The red container is for disposing of infectious plastics like urine bags, blood bags and catheters. The black container is for disposing of expired drugs and radioactive substances.

3. (A) Encourage patients to wash their hands before using the toilet.

Handwashing before using the toilet doesn't reduce the risk of hospital-acquired urinary tract infections. Preventive measures to reduce hospital-acquired urinary tract infections include avoidance of invasive urethral procedures like catheterization, prevention of urine stasis, increased urine output and use of prophylactic antibiotics.

4. (B) Face masks are used for contact isolation measures.

Face masks aren't used for contact isolation measures because the contact route of transmission doesn't involve aerosols and droplet nuclei. Gloves, gowns and boots are used for contact isolation measures.

5. (B) Air flows out of the room but not into it.

Negative pressure rooms have a lower pressure compared to their surroundings. As a result, the air is sucked and trapped into the room but doesn't flow out. Examples of negative pressure rooms are isolation rooms to isolate clients with airborne infections like SARS.

6. (D) Autopsy rooms have positive pressure.

Autopsy rooms actually have negative pressure. Negative pressure rooms are designed to allow inflow of air but not outflow. Rooms with positive pressure are designed to permit air outflow but not inflow. Examples of rooms with positive room pressure are operating rooms.

7. (C) 9.

This child has an Apgar score of 9.

Appearance – pink trunk with blue extremities (1)

Pulse greater than 100 bpm (2)

Cries with stimulation (2)

Active, spontaneous movement (2)

Good cry (2)

8. (A) Suction the nostrils with a suction bulb.

This child needs mild suctioning of his airway to improve breathing. Option B is incorrect because the child's heart rate is greater than 100 bpm. Options C and D are incorrect because CPAP and IV epinephrine are indicated for neonates with birth asphyxia.

9. (D) Disulfiram is the antidote of choice.

Disulfiram is used to treat alcoholism. Disulfiram inhibits the enzymatic action of acetaldehyde dehydrogenase. The buildup of acetaldehyde causes unpleasant hangover effects. Acetylcysteine (Mucomyst) is the antidote of choice for acetaminophen poisoning. Acetylcysteine replenishes the diminished glutathione reserves in the liver and reduces the risk of acute liver failure.

10. (C) DIC.

DIC is a common feature of meningococcemia, which is caused by *Neisseria meningitides*. Meningococcemia occurs about 24–48 hours after *N. meningitides* infection and is characterized by diffused vascular injury, circulatory shock and DIC. Epilepsy, deafness and hydrocephalus are all chronic complications of meningitis. Acute complications include DIC, SIADH, seizures, cerebral edema and raised intracranial pressure.

11. (C) If the baby has pink skin and blue extremities, he is given a score of 1 for appearance.

Option A is incorrect because an Apgar score is given to a neonate in the first and fifth minute of life. Option B is incorrect because a pulse rate that is less than 100 bpm has a score of 1. Option D is incorrect because a grimace has a score of 1.

12. (D) Giving a surfactant.

The use of surfactants is not indicated in this term neonate. Also, a surfactant is not used as an emergency measure for hypoxia. Useful measures to stimulate respiration in neonates include drying, rubbing of the child's back and feet, suctioning of the airway and using assistive ventilation devices.

13. (D) Obtaining parental consent for contraception.

Parental consent is usually not needed for providing contraceptives to a sexually active teenager. However, this client will benefit from measures that will reduce her chances of getting pregnant and contracting an STI.

14. (B) 10%.

In severe dehydration, at least 10–15% of the body's water is lost. In moderate dehydration, about 6–10% of the water volume is lost. In mild dehydration, less than 5% of the body's water is lost. Severe dehydration is an emergency and a common cause of hypovolemic shock. Other causes of severe dehydration include burns, diabetic ketoacidosis, hyperpyrexia and kidney failure.

15. (A) 10% dextrose water.

Hypoglycemic infants lack the necessary glucose needed for metabolism. 10% dextrose water has the appropriate amount of glucose needed. The other fluids are contraindicated in the management of hypoglycemia. Ringer's lactate is used for severe hypokalemia and acute resuscitation. The dextrose in 4.3% and 5% dextrose saline isn't adequate for resuscitation and maintenance. Also, the kidneys of a newborn are not yet mature enough to handle the solute salts in these fluids.

16. (C) Potassium.

Severe vomiting is a usual symptom of intestinal obstruction. Potassium isn't lost significantly through vomiting. However, large losses of hydrogen ions in the vomitus can trigger metabolic alkalosis. In this case, post-emetic bicarbonaturia can induce heavy losses of potassium ions in the urine.

17. (D) Calcium gluconate.

Although calcium gluconate is part of the management guidelines for hyperkalemia, it doesn't reduce potassium levels in the blood. Rather, it increases the threshold potential of cardiac muscles, stabilizing the resting membrane potential and reducing the incidence of arrhythmia and cardiac arrest. Insulin and salbutamol drive potassium into the cells. Cation exchange resins increase potassium through the gut and are useful for clients with poor urine output.

18. (C) There is destruction of the alpha cells in the pancreas.

Type 1 diabetes mellitus is an autoimmune disease of the pancreas. The beta cells of the pancreas are destroyed by the body's antibodies by mediating a Type IV hypersensitivity reaction. In this case, there is an activation of T-helper cells, CD8 cells and the innate immune system. The treatment of choice is insulin, which is used for life.

19. (B) Acetylcholine.

Antidepressants are based on the monoamine hypothesis which states that depression is caused by an imbalance of monoamine neurotransmitters like serotonin, norepinephrine and dopamine. Acetylcholine is not a monoamine. It is an ester of choline and acetic acid, which is produced in the parasympathetic nervous system. Myasthenia gravis is a disorder of acetylcholine signal transmission at the motor endplate.

20. (D) Jaundice.

Jaundice is not a likely feature of peptic ulcer disease. Features of peptic ulcer disease include signs and symptoms of upper gastrointestinal bleeding, bloating, epigastric pain, vomiting and changes in bowel habits.

Jaundice is a clinical feature of impaired excretion of bilirubin caused by an increased bilirubin production and impaired bilirubin metabolism and excretion.

21. (B) Rye.

Gluten is a group of proteins present in cereal grains like wheat, spelt and rye. These proteins give these cereal grains a glue-like consistency when they are ground into flour and mixed with water. These proteins also give dough its characteristic chewy and elastic texture. Clients with gluten intolerance produce antibodies that attack the antigens in gluten.

22. (C) Ergosterol.

Ergosterol is a derivative of vitamin D, a fat-soluble vitamin. Alcoholics have reduced amounts of vitamin B complexes and vitamin A. However, vitamin D deficiency is less likely in this case because these are more prevalent in clients who don't receive sufficient sunlight. Other causes of vitamin D deficiency include but are not limited to renal diseases, liver diseases and malabsorption syndrome.

23. (D) Vitamin K.

Metabolism of vitamin K occurs in the colon, where gut flora converts vitamin K1 into vitamin K2. Folic acid and iron absorption occur at lower pH (acidic) levels. Zinc absorption is impaired by intestinal surgeries such as gastric bypass surgery.

24. (D) Monitor for constipation.

Clients with end-stage hepatic failure are at risk for hepatic encephalopathy. In such cases, ammonia accumulates in the blood, passes through the blood-brain barrier and destroys neurons. To prevent this, clients with decompensated liver failure are monitored to prevent the accumulation of ammonia. Some of these strategies include reduction of protein intake, prevention of constipation and enhanced excretion of ammonia. The use of sedatives is contraindicated in their management because it can mask an ongoing encephalopathy. TPN isn't beneficial unless indicated.

25. (D) A client with hemorrhoids.

Melena stools are a sign of upper gastrointestinal bleeding. Blood tracks down the gut and comes out in the feces as altered dark blood with a characteristic odor. All the clients listed above are likely to have upper GI bleeding except the client with hemorrhoids, who has lower GI bleeding. This client is likely to pass fresh blood in his stool. Causes of upper GI bleeding include peptic ulcer disease, upper GI tumors and Mallory–Weiss tears.

26. (A) It's a precancerous state.

Gynecomastia is an increase in the size of male breast tissue. It is caused by an imbalance in the estrogen/androgen ratio. Causes include chronic kidney and liver diseases that impair metabolism and excretion of sex hormones; estrogen-secreting tumors of the lungs, adrenals and testes; certain drugs and chronic alcohol consumption. Gynecomastia is not a precancerous state, although most clients worry that it is.

27. (C) Bacterial vaginosis.

Bacterial vaginosis is a vaginal tract infection caused by the overgrowth of opportunistic vaginal flora. Symptoms include watery yellow or green discharge with a characteristic fishy odor, burning sensation upon urination and itching. Some clients may be asymptomatic. Bacterial vaginosis increases the rate of transmission of HIV and other STIs.

28. (C) Gardasil 9 can be given to older people.

Option A is incorrect because Gardasil 9 prevents infection from carcinogenic strains of HPV 16 and 18. Option B is incorrect because the vaccine is given to both prepubertal boys and girls of ages 11–12, although vaccines can be given as early as age 9. It can also be given to older people, as long as they haven't been infected by HPV 16 and 18. Option D is incorrect because the Gardasil 9 vaccine doesn't protect from STIs.

29. (B) Secondary infertility.

A couple is said to have secondary infertility when either one or both partners have achieved conception before. Primary infertility occurs when neither of the partners has achieved conception before. Options C and D are incorrect because although chronic PID and hypogonadism are causes of infertility, there is no clinical information that confirms these diagnoses.

30. (D) Unintentional weight loss.

Polycystic ovarian syndrome is an endocrine disorder of females caused by high levels of androgens. Features of PCOS include but are not limited to scanty, heavy or absent menstrual periods, hirsutism, acne and infertility. It is usually associated with type 2 diabetes, obesity, obstructive sleep apnea and heart disease.

31. (A) 39°C – hyperpyrexia.

Hyperpyrexia is a temperature of 41°C and above. It is a life-threatening occurrence.

32. (C) Colostomy irrigation.

Colostomy irrigation is a septic procedure.

33. (C) It can be formal or standardized.

Nursing care plans can either be formal or informal plans. Formal plans can either be standardized or individualized.

34. (A) The position of the bed.

Prayer is a core value in a Muslim's life. A Muslim prays facing the direction of the Kaaba in Mecca. Positioning the bed in relation to the direction of the Kaaba will help the Muslim patient observe his religious duties.

35. (C) Roasted chicken and vegetable fried rice.

Eating kosher is a religious and cultural food tradition for the Jews. Some aspects of this tradition restrict Jews from eating seafood without scales (shrimp, lobster, snails, clams) and also from eating dairy and meat in the same dish. It also restricts Jews from eating non-ruminant animals. Option A is incorrect because it contains seafood without scales. Option B is incorrect because it contains dairy and beef. Option D is incorrect because it contains meat from a non-ruminant animal.

36. (B) Forming a plan of action.

In this technique, the listener attempts to make the speaker aware of other existing options. Unlike the non-therapeutic technique of giving advice, this technique is non-confrontational and non-evaluative.

37. (A) When did this start?

The therapeutic communication technique of placing the event in time or sequence helps the speaker to understand the chronology of the speaker's challenge. However, this technique uses open-ended questions that enable the speaker to speak freely.

38. (D) "I see that you regret your actions."

Option A is incorrect because it is an example of the non-therapeutic technique of giving advice. Option B is incorrect because it is an example of the non-therapeutic technique of giving false reassurances. Option C is incorrect because it is an example of the non-therapeutic technique of probing.

39. (B) Giving false reassurances.

This technique is non-therapeutic because by informing the client that there is no cause for worry or alarm, the nurse is conveying that he/she regards the client's worry as invalid.

40. (B) Presenting reality.

This technique involves the use of direct statements of facts to the client. This technique blocks communication because the client may feel threatened and may refuse to communicate further.

41. (D) Health insurance fraud.

Criminal acts deal with acts that are illegal. These include felony and misdemeanor acts like falsifying medical records, practicing without a license, practicing with an expired license, stealing and abuse of drugs.

42. (B) Civil.

Civil law focuses on disputes between people. This law addresses the legal rights of patients and the responsibilities of nurses to their patients.

43. (A) Administrative law.

Administrative law includes the rules and regulations that support statutory law established by a legislative body.

44. (B) Blood pressure measurement.

Nursing assistants work under the supervision of an RN to provide personalized care to clients. Some of the services nursing assistants provide include monitoring of vital signs, assistance with dressing, eating, bathing and walking.

Vaginal examinations, monitoring uterine contractions and oxytocin administration should be performed by a midwife or an obstetrician.

45. (B) Administer IV antibiotics.

LPNs are skilled in performing practical tasks like measuring vital signs, administering medications and helping clients eat, dress and bathe. However, analytical skills are done by an RN.

46. (C) Stop the blood transfusion immediately.

Anaphylactic reactions occur when antibodies mount an immune response to certain antigens which act as allergens. These reactions are sudden in onset, severe and life-threatening. Symptoms of anaphylactic reactions include but are not limited to hypotension, fever, itching, rashes and swelling of soft tissues. Anaphylaxis is managed symptomatically using vasoconstrictors, antihistamines and steroids. But the priority response is to remove the offending allergen as quickly as possible.

47. (A) Use a medication compatibility chart.

A medication compatibility chart reduces the incidence of IV drug incompatibility by providing quick information on the compatibility of various IV drugs and IV fluids. These charts not only prevent harmful drug interactions but also save time and prevent waste of drugs.

48. (B) Vastus lateralis.

The vastus lateralis is part of the muscles of the anterior thigh. IM medications are given at the bulkiest part of the vastus, to prevent nerve and blood vessel damage. Options A and C are incorrect because the gluteus maximus and deltoid muscle are underdeveloped in neonates and are not ideal sites for administration. The gluteus maximus is generally avoided to prevent damage to the sciatic nerve. Option D is incorrect because the biceps are not a safe site for IM medications because of their relation to the brachial artery and the brachial plexus.

49. (D) Ringer's lactate.

In gastroenteritis, there is ongoing potassium loss. A dextrose infusion will cause more potassium loss because glucose stimulates insulin secretion. Insulin causes a shift in potassium from plasma into the cells. Ringer's lactate contains potassium and is therefore suitable for use. Apart from Ringer's, 0.9% normal saline can also be used.

50. (B) Normal saline.

A patient with diabetic ketoacidosis is severely dehydrated (about 10% water loss). About 6–8 L of normal saline is used in acute resuscitation. Dextrose water and dextrose saline are contraindicated because they contain glucose and will worsen the acidosis. Ringer's lactate, which contains potassium, isn't indicated. However, intravenous potassium can be added into the normal saline after the commencement of insulin.

51. (D) Implantable ports are not indicated for cachectic and obese patients.

Option A is incorrect because peripherally inserted central lines are either inserted in the cephalic vein or basilic vein. Option B is incorrect because centrally non-tunneled central lines are also called Hickman Lines. Option C is incorrect because implantable ports are contraindicated for obese and cachectic clients.

52. (A) Omalizumab.

Omalizumab is a monoclonal antibody that binds to both free and membrane-bound IgE. This action inhibits Type 1 immediate hypersensitivity reactions that occur in urticaria. However, Omalizumab is not beneficial for acute episodes of urticaria because it doesn't bind to IgE that is bound to mast cells, basophils and dendritic cells. This property makes it unsuitable for acute treatment but ideal for preventing future reactions.

53. (A) Pyridoxine.

Isoniazid is associated with pyridoxine (vitamin B6) deficiency because Isoniazid, which has the same structure as pyridoxine, competes for the same enzyme needed in pyridoxine metabolism. Isoniazid also increases the excretion of pyridoxine. Pyridoxine deficiency causes sideroblastic anemia.

54. (C) Cobalamin supplements.

Vitamin B12, which is also known as cobalamin, is not a cause of drug-induced paresthesia. However, paresthesia can be caused by vitamin B5 and vitamin B12 deficiencies. Nitrofurantoin, isoniazid and phenytoin are causes of drug-induced paresthesia. Vitamin B5 and B12 supplements are prescribed along with these drugs to reduce the risk of drug-induced paresthesia.

55. (B) Step 1 involves the use of diclofenac with or without adjuvants.

Step 1 involves the use of non-opioid drugs like NSAIDs and acetaminophen with or without the use of adjuvants. Step 1 is used for mild pain, graded 1–4. Examples of adjuvants include sedatives and immunosuppressors like prednisolone.

56. (C) Hydrocodone.

Hydrocodone is a weak opioid agonist. Other weak agonists include codeine and dihydrocodeine. Strong opioid agonists include morphine, hydromorphone, fentanyl and pethidine, among all the other answers listed.

57. (B) It is an opioid antagonist.

Naltrexone is an opioid antagonist that is indicated in an overdose of opioid drugs. Side effects of Naltrexone include nausea, vomiting, dizziness, headaches and withdrawal symptoms.

58. (C) Intratracheal.

A surfactant is given through a catheter passed through the neonate's endotracheal tube. It is not given through any other means.

59. (A) A 58-year-old woman with fibroids.

Estrogen is implicated in fibroids and is, therefore, contraindicated in this client. Risk factors of fibroids include early menarche, late childbearing and infertility, all of which indicate high estrogenic states. Estrogen therapy is indicated for dysfunctional uterine bleeding, post-menopausal syndrome and primary hypogonadism.

60. (B) A normal respiratory rate.

The respiratory rate of a six-year-old ranges from 12 to 30 cycles per minute. Option D is incorrect because crepitations are assessed during auscultation and not during an inspection.

61. (B) A laryngoscope.

You don't need a laryngoscope to view the tonsils. A laryngoscope is used to view the larynx. The laryngoscope is used for more complex procedures like removing foreign bodies stuck in the throat, assessing the airway for cancerous growths and collecting tissues for biopsies.

62. (D) A client who has undergone hip replacement surgery.

Pelvic surgery is a strong risk factor for deep vein thrombosis. Although the other clients are at risk of developing DVT, there isn't enough clinical history to suggest they have the greatest risk.

63. (B) ALP.

Cardiac markers are enzymatic biomarkers used to evaluate heart function. Examples include troponin, CK MB, LDH, AST and myoglobin. ALP is an enzyme marker used to assess liver function.

64. (C) An elderly client with metastatic CAP to the lumbar vertebrae.

Orthostatic pneumonia occurs when there is pooling and stagnation of fluid in the lungs. This form of pneumonia is common in elderly and bedridden clients. This client is most at risk because he is bedridden due to the metastatic spread of prostate cancer to his lumbar vertebrae.

65. (D) Dubin–Johnson Syndrome.

Dubin–Johnson Syndrome is a cause of conjugated hyperbilirubinemia. It is a benign genetic disorder characterized by conjugated bilirubinemia, dark liver and chromosomal defect of protein carriers. Usually, there is no treatment because this disease is benign, with no morbidity or mortality. This form of jaundice is not treatable with phototherapy. Phototherapy is used for managing unconjugated hyperbilirubinemia. All the other options are causes of unconjugated bilirubinemia.

66. (A) Jaundice from the fourth day of life.

Pathologic jaundice occurs from the first day of life and persists until medical intervention is done. Physiologic jaundice occurs from the second to the fourth day of life and fades by the second week. It is caused by rapid lysis of fragile red blood cells and an inability of the neonate's growing liver to efficiently conjugate and excrete bilirubin.

67. (D) Respiratory rate.

Respiratory rate is not a factor for measuring dehydration status in children. Useful factors include pulse, blood pressure, skin turgidity, buccal mucosa, eyes, fontanelle, capillary refill and level of consciousness.

68. (D) Sclera.

The sclera is the white part of the eye. It is avascular and therefore can't be used to assess pallor. Pallor is assessed on vascularized tissues like the buccal mucosa, conjunctiva, palms and soles. The sclera is used to assess jaundice.

69. (A) Petechiae rash.

Petechiae rashes are small purple-red rashes on the skin surface. They are caused by bleeding from a broken capillary vessel. A common cause is a bleeding disorder from coagulopathies. These rashes are non-blanchable.

Erythema is a redness of the skin due to hyperthermia. Malar rashes occur in the face, and miliaria is also known as heat rash.

70. (C) Orthostatic pneumonia.

Orthostatic pneumonia is common in the elderly and bedridden patients. The lungs are congested with blood, which promotes the growth and proliferation of infectious bacteria. There is no clinical history that suggests that this client is bedridden.

71. (C) Urolithiasis.

Also known as kidney stones, urolithiasis is the accumulation of precipitated salts and calculi in the kidneys or any other part of the urinary tract. Risk factors for kidney stones include hypercalcemia, hyperuricemia, dehydration, obstructive uropathy and certain drugs. This client has hypoproteinemia, which is not a risk factor for kidney stones.

72. (B) Provide muscle physiotherapy.

The absence of movement against gravity and resistance in a bedridden patient causes muscles to atrophy from disuse.

Regular physiotherapy can increase muscle bulk by putting stress and strain on muscles and joints.

73. (C) Turning the client from left, right and back every two hours to relieve pressure.

Option A is incorrect because linen layers increase friction and shearing. Option B is incorrect because skin assessments are done every eight hours. Option D is incorrect because lubrication with oily or water-based substances is strongly discouraged. Part of the nursing interventions for bedridden clients is to keep pressure areas dry and moisture-free.

74. (D) Reverse Trendelenburg position.

This position provides quick relief to patients by increasing gastric motility and preventing the reflux of gastric contents.

Options A and B are incorrect because the High Fowler's and Low Fowler's positions are used to improve respiration and relieve respiratory distress. Option C is incorrect because the lithotomy position is used for vaginal examinations and childbirth.

75. (B) Malabsorption.

Malabsorption is not a problem of the oral and nasal cavities but of the intestines. In this condition, there is an impaired absorption of food nutrients. Children with cleft palates have problems in the oral and nasal cavity.

76. (A) A client who had a craniotomy for cerebral hemorrhage.

This position will improve cerebral venous drainage and reduce the risk of raised cranial pressure. The clients with herniorrhaphy and spinal anesthesia will benefit from a supine position. The client who had the liver biopsy will benefit from a left lateral position.

77. (B) A client who is one-hour post-op from an arterio-vascular graft.

This client needs to be on bed rest for at least 24 hours to encourage uptake of the graft.

78. (B) Eat highly fatty foods to improve bile secretion.

Fatty foods can increase gastric acid secretion and worsen reflux. This client should be counseled to eat less fatty foods to get relief.

79. (B) Pyrexia – cold water bath.

Tepid water, not cold water, is used for clients with pyrexia. Cold water will lower the client's temperature too quickly and cause chills.

80. (B) Denial.

In denial, the affected person refuses to admit to a painful reality. Reality is often treated as if it is not real.

81. (B) Projection.

In projection, the affected person blames others for his feelings and actions.

82. (A) Social model of disability.

The social model focuses on the attitudes and systemic biases that make it hard for clients with disabilities to attain functionality. Option B is incorrect because the biomedical model focuses on treating and managing disabilities. Option C is incorrect because the cognitive model focuses on improving the existing abilities of a client with a disability. Option D is incorrect because the term "biosocial model of disability" is fictitious.

83. (A) Treating and managing disabilities.

This method is focused on treating and managing disabilities. It is not focused on primary prevention methods of disabilities and is also not the basis of the social model of disability.

84. (A) Responding to his own name.

Developmental milestones in a six-month-old include an ability to respond to his name, recognize familiar faces, respond to sounds by making sounds, string vowels together when babbling and bring things to his mouth.

Options B and D are incorrect because an ability to follow instructions and make sentences with two to four words is a developmental milestone for two-year-olds. Option C is incorrect because an ability to stand with support is a developmental milestone for a 10-month-old child.

85. (D) Telling stories.

A two-year-old has motor and cognitive functions that are complex but not yet varied. The child can engage in simple tasks like pointing to things in a book, knocking down a block of building towers and following simple instructions. Complex functions like telling stories are milestones achieved by four-year-olds.

86. (C) A 75-year-old female with Alzheimer's disease.

Clients at risk of elder abuse are often women with mental and cognitive impairments that make them more dependent and vulnerable to their caregivers. They usually stay alone or with the caregiver. It is known that women are at risk of persistent and severe forms of abuse.

87. (B) Overgrown nails.

Premature babies are small and have a disproportionately large head. They have little fat stores and underdeveloped genitalia. They have shiny pink skin that can be translucent with lanugo hair. Overgrown nails are features found in post-term babies born after 40 weeks.

88. (A) Diminished vesicular breath sounds can indicate COPD.

Bronchial sounds are abnormal findings. A bronchial breath is a high-pitched sound heard when normal lung tissue is replaced by fibrosed tissue that has an underlying latent bronchus.

Options C and D are incorrect because breath sounds are loudest at the apex in early inspiration and loudest at the base in mid-inspiration.

89. (C) S1 is loud at the apex and S2 is faint at the base.

S1 is caused by the closure of the mitral and tricuspid valves, and it is best heard at the apex. S2, which is heard by the closure of the pulmonary and aortic valves, is best heard at the base/left parasternal edge.

90. (A) A positive fluid thrill.

A fluid thrill is an examination done on the anterior abdominal wall to assess ascites. A positive fluid thrill is detected in gross ascites, which are typically found in decompensated liver disease. Shifting dullness is used to assess moderate ascites.

91. (C) Hydronephrosis.

In a renal examination, healthy kidneys are not easily ballotable except for the inferior pole of the right kidney. An easily palpable kidney can have an underlying inflammatory process that changes the structural integrity of the renal medulla and capsule. Hydronephrosis is also known as edema of the kidneys. It can be caused by obstructive uropathy or an inflammatory process.

92. (A) Scrub your hands for at least 10 seconds.

The correct duration for handwashing is 15–20 seconds. Kids are encouraged to time themselves by singing the “Happy Birthday” song at least twice.

93. (C) Hepatitis B – from birth.

Options A, C and D are all incorrect because the first doses of these vaccines are given from eight weeks.

94. (D) Tetanus vaccine.

The tetanus vaccine is a toxoid vaccine. Toxoid vaccines are produced from toxins released from certain bacteria. This protein-based toxin is inactivated and used as an antigen to elicit active artificial immunity. The diphtheria vaccine is an example of a toxoid vaccine.

95. (B) Polycythemia.

This infant is premature. All of the answer options are common complications of prematurity except polycythemia. A premature infant is at risk of anemia.

96. (B) A high whey content.

The protein content in breast milk is about 60% whey and 40% casein. Its high whey content makes it easily digestible by infants. Infant formulas have a high casein content and aren't easily digested compared to whey. Options C and D are incorrect because bifidus factor and IgA contribute to the immune-boosting properties of milk.

97. (B) A five-year-old male with a history of intussusception.

Clients with a history of intussusception or combined immunodeficiency disease are not eligible for a rotavirus vaccine.

98. (D) Phototherapy.

Kangaroo mother care is used for premature and hospitalized neonates for warmth, bonding and breastfeeding. It is not used to provide phototherapy. Phototherapy, using a phototherapy machine, is given to neonates who are jaundiced.

99. (B) Handwashing.

Hepatitis A is spread by direct contact with contaminated feces.

100. (D) Impaired bile acid excretion.

In obstructive jaundice, there is an obstruction to the outflow and excretion of bile acids.

Answers to Test 3

1. (D) Hypothermia.

This neonate is macrosomic. He has a large body surface area and larger than normal amounts of somatic cells and fat cells. Hypothermia is not a likely complication.

2. (D) Weight gain.

Weight gain is a common side effect of hormonal contraceptives. Copper IUDs do not contain any hormones.

3. (C) IgA – supports the growth of lactobacillus.

IgA confers passive immunity to viral and bacterial infections of the gut and respiratory tract. It doesn't support the growth of lactobacillus. Bifidus factor supports the growth of lactobacillus.

4. (A) Chlamydia.

Prophylactic chloramphenicol and erythromycin are put into the eyes of newborns to prevent eye infections caused by gonorrhea and chlamydia.

5. (D) Neonatal jaundice.

This client has gestational diabetes. Neonatal jaundice is a neonatal complication of gestational diabetes and not a maternal complication.

6. (A) Scabies.

Scabies is a parasitic skin infestation spread through close contact and indirect contact from fomites like clothes and bedsheets. Handwashing does not prevent scabies. Prevention of scabies includes washing and sun-drying of clothes as well as prevention of overcrowding and sharing of personal effects.

7. (C) Wash and store all clothes in airtight bags for at least 48 hours.

A primary prevention method is to wash and sun-dry all clothes then store them in airtight containers for at least 48 hours to suffocate the ticks.

8. (C) Cervical insufficiency.

Cervical insufficiency is a cause of first trimester miscarriages. In this condition, the cervix effaces and dilates before the onset of labor. Most causes of cervical insufficiency are congenital and non-modifiable.

9. (B) This client has a physical dependence on nicotine use.

A client is said to have a physical dependence when he suffers adverse and unwanted physical and physiological effects when he stops taking the drug. The symptoms of nicotine withdrawal include nausea, abdominal pain, constipation, sweating, tingling sensation in the feet and arms, headaches and insomnia.

10. (C) Systemic desensitization.

In systemic desensitization, the client is exposed to an increasing dose of fear-provoking stimulus for desensitization. This provoking stimulus is paired with a relaxing stimulus.

11. (B) Group therapy.

Group therapy is beneficial for clients with personality disorders. These clients do well in a group of people who face similar challenges. In these groups, participants are free to express their feelings and they are offered practical help and support.

12. (A) Concrete thinking.

Teenagers are abstract thinkers. They show an increasing interest in aesthetic and philosophical values. These values form a basis for their personalities, convictions and habits. Four-year-olds think concretely and are unable to differentiate the real from the imagined.

13. (D) Monitor vital signs, electrolytes and blood gases.

This client is at risk of developing severe and life-threatening complications caused by imbalances in electrolytes, blood gases and nutrients. These imbalances put the client at risk of complications like arrhythmia, hypokalemia, severe dehydration, refeeding syndrome, hypothermia and hypoglycemia.

14. (C) The child refuses to make eye contact with the examiner.

Since the health worker is a strange and unfamiliar face, the child may not be comfortable making eye contact. This is a normal response for his age.

15. (C) Ensure the safety of the child.

The safety of this child is paramount. Before doing anything else, you should ensure that the child is in a safe environment and away from further harm.

16. (A) An environment that is familiar and routine.

An autistic child is not comfortable with change. A familiar environment with routine activities assures the child. It also reduces episodes, tantrums and meltdowns.

17. (D) Debriding the wound with a surgical laser.

This client has a fresh ulcer that needs to be covered and protected from superseding infection. Surgical debridement is not indicated because the wound is not necrotic.

18. (C) Maintaining a slow infusion rate to prevent overfeeding and diarrhea.

Option A is incorrect because clients on nasogastric tube feeding are at risk of diarrhea and not constipation. Option B is incorrect because increased water intake is not indicated for this client since he's not on a urethral catheter. Option D is incorrect because daily turning isn't indicated since the client is not bedridden.

19. (D) High-protein diet to prevent muscle atrophy.

This intervention is not indicated because although cancer is a catabolic state, a high protein diet may not only be unnecessary, but harmful. A balanced diet, a healthy appetite and regular exercise are useful in maintaining an optimal weight.

20. (C) Encourage the client to eat small, frequent meals.

Option A is incorrect because a nasogastric tube can be uncomfortable for a fully conscious patient. Option B is incorrect because a dextrose infusion isn't indicated unless the client is hypoglycemic. Option D is incorrect because spicy foods can increase the risk of gastritis and reflux disease.

21. (C) Remove old ties before securing new ones.

New ties are secured before removing old ones. This is done to prevent the dislodgement of the tracheostomy tube.

22. (D) Use a therapeutic communication technique.

This client is anxious about the surgery. Therapeutic communication may be all that is needed to calm her down. If it fails, other interventions can be considered. Option A is incorrect because you need a doctor's order before giving an anxiolytic.

23. (C) Stop solid food by 12 a.m., then the child can drink breast milk till 2 a.m. and can drink clear fluids till 6 a.m.

Children are at risk for dehydration, so adequate hydration is necessary. Babies and toddlers between the ages of six months and three years can eat solid foods until eight hours before surgery. They can drink milk, formula or breast milk until six hours before surgery. Children can drink clear fluids until two hours before surgery.

24. (C) Yogurt.

Yogurt is not a clear fluid and cannot be consumed less than six hours before surgery. Clear fluids like water, apple juice, cranberry juice and electrolyte-replenishing drinks can be consumed two hours before surgery.

25. (C) End-stage renal disease.

Also known as Ringer's lactate, Hartmann's solution contains potassium. Potassium is required in conditions where there is ongoing potassium loss, such as in intestinal obstruction and pancreatitis. Hartmann's is also used for resuscitation in patients with burn injuries. A client with end-stage renal disease is at risk of having hyperkalemia, not hypokalemia.

26. (C) 21 gtt/min

The formula for drop rate is $\frac{volume \times dropfactor}{time}$

Volume = 500 ml

Drop factor = 20 gtt/ml

Time (minutes) = 8 × 60 = 480 minutes

Drop rate = $\frac{500ml \times 20gtt/ml}{480\,\text{min}}$

Drop rate = 20.83 gtt/min = 21 gtt/min.

27. (B) 25 gtt/min.

The formula for drop rate is $\frac{volume \times dropfactor}{time}$

Volume = 150 ml

Drop factor of a soluset = 60 gtt/ml

Time (minutes) = 6 × 60 = 360 minutes

Drop rate = $\frac{150ml \times 60gtt / ml}{360\,\text{min}}$

Drop rate = 25 gtt/min

28. (B) As an intravenous infusion.

Vancomycin is given slowly over 60 minutes as an intravenous infusion. Option A is incorrect because a rapid administration as a bolus can cause flushing, pruritus and erythema. This is called red man syndrome. Rapid administration can also cause hypotension and urticaria. Option C is incorrect because vancomycin is a tissue irritant and is not given via an intramuscular route. Option D is incorrect because it is given as an oral capsule.

29. (D) Metronidazole – diarrhea.

Common adverse effects of metronidazole include nausea, vomiting, diarrhea, abdominal pain, dizziness and a metallic taste in the mouth. Option A is incorrect because streptomycin can cause deafness. Option B is incorrect because tetracycline causes teeth discoloration in children. Option C is incorrect because isoniazid causes paresthesia.

30. (A) 18G.

Size 16G and 18G cannulae are preferred for obstetric patients in labor. The width, length and flow rates of these cannulas are ideal for rapid blood transfusion and intravenous infusions. The features of these cannulae are suitable for obstetric clients because these clients have a risk of hemorrhage and dehydration and will need acute resuscitation with either blood or intravenous fluids.

31. (D) Placenta previa.

Placenta previa, which is the abnormal location of the placenta at the internal os, is a life-threatening cause of antepartum hemorrhage. Vaginal delivery is contra-indicated. Women with placenta previa can have elective caesarean sections at 38 weeks.

32. (D) Ondansetron.

Ondansetron is a serotonin receptor antagonist. It is used to treat chemotherapy-induced vomiting. Its side effects include diarrhea, constipation, headache and dizziness. The other options are all chemotherapeutic drugs with vomiting as a side effect.

33. (D) Dexamethasone.

Although dexamethasone is indicated in preterm labor, it's beneficial because it stimulates the maturation of the fetus' lungs. The other drugs listed are tocolytics, which relax the uterine muscle.

34. (D) Chloroquine.

All the drugs listed above are implicated in Stevens–Johnson, a Type IV hypersensitivity reaction of the skin. These drugs include certain antiretrovirals, antihypertensives and a broad class of sulfonamides.

35. (C) Faces pain rating scale.

The faces pain rating scale is ideal for children who are unable to describe their pain using verbal or numerical indices. Indices used for the faces pain rating scale include smiling, frowning, crying, etc.

36. (C) Diabetes mellitus.

This client has hypoalbuminemia. Diabetes mellitus is not a cause of hypoalbuminemia. It is a metabolic disorder of nutrient metabolism. It is also characterized by excessive catabolism of glycogen, protein and fatty acids to yield energy.

37. (D) Thrombocytopenia.

Although malignant hypertension can cause coagulopathies, it doesn't affect the number of platelets. The client is at risk of developing all the other complications listed in the answer choices.

38. (A) Withhold the next dose of warfarin.

A patient on warfarin is at risk of developing coagulopathies. To reduce this risk, the clotting profile of the client is constantly monitored. The normal PT is 9.6–11.8 secs. This client has increased bleeding time and is at risk of developing a bleeding disorder. Therefore, the next dose of warfarin should be withheld.

39. (C) This test is diagnostic of neural tube defects.

Alpha-fetoprotein is used to diagnose neural tube defects. Amniocentesis is then done to confirm the diagnosis. Option A is incorrect because chromosomal abnormalities are diagnosed with HCG. Options B and D are incorrect because alpha-fetoprotein isn't diagnostic of lung and cardiac disorders.

40. (D) Diarrhea.

A bedridden patient is at risk of constipation. Because the client is immobile, there is a breakdown and release of excess calcium from the bones. This hypercalcemia causes constipation. Also, immobility reduces blood flow to the gastrointestinal tract. This causes reduced motile function and constipation.

41. (A) This client has rheumatoid arthritis.

This client has gouty arthritis, an accumulation of uric acid precipitates in joints. The risk factors of gouty arthritis include obesity, alcohol intake, consumption of red meat, seafood and other foods that are high in purines. Treatment includes the use of NSAIDs and allopurinol.

42. (D) Metabolic acidosis.

This client's bicarbonate ions are reduced. Also, his urea and creatinine are increased due to impaired renal function. He needs urgent hemodialysis. In end-stage renal disease, there is inefficient ammonia excretion and reduced tubular reabsorption of bicarbonate. All these contribute to metabolic acidosis.

43. (D) Respiratory alkalosis.

This client is suffering from hyperventilation. As a result, there is increased respiration, increased gaseous exchange of carbon dioxide for oxygen and consequent washing out of carbon dioxide from the bloodstream.

44. (B) Twin gestation.

Twin gestation is not an absolute indication for a caesarean section. A woman with a twin gestation can be allowed to have a vaginal delivery unless there are certain risk factors like abnormal lie and presentation of the leading twin.

45. (A) From the tip of the nose to the earlobe to the xiphisternum.

The nasogastric tube is inserted through the pharynx and right into the gastroesophageal junction. This is roughly measured from the tip of the nose to the earlobe to the xiphisternum.

46. (B) The chest tube is draining actively.

Continuous bubbling in the suction chamber means that the drain is working. Intermittent bubbling means that there is a block in the tube. A dislodged tube is uncomfortable for a client. The client can complain of pain.

47. (D) A client with a lumbar puncture.

The client with a lumbar puncture should be in a supine position for at least five hours. This posture prevents the risk of rapid redistribution of CSF and subsequent headaches.

48. (B) Frontal lobe.

Broca's area is the speech center located in the frontal lobe of the cerebral cortex. When this area is affected by a thrombotic or ischemic CVD, clients become aphasic. Option A is incorrect because an infarct in the occipital lobe can cause visual disorders like complete blindness, visual hallucinations and visual syndromes. Option C is incorrect because an infarct in the parietal lobe can cause upper and lower limb weakness. Option D is incorrect because the sagittal lobe is a fictitious term.

49. (B) 4.

The Glasgow Coma Scale (GCS) is used to assess head injuries by using parameters that measure eye, motor and verbal response. A GCS score of 13 or above indicates a minor head injury. A score of 9 to 12 indicates a moderate head injury. Severe head injuries have a score that ranges from 3–8.

50. (B) 5.

The client had the best eye response of 1, the best motor response of 2 and the best verbal response of 2.

51. (C) Vitamin C metabolism.

Vitamin C is a water-soluble vitamin that can only be sourced exogenously from fruits, vegetables and other food sources. Gut bacteria haven't been shown to improve the synthesis and absorption of vitamin C.

52. (A) Copper IUD.

This client will benefit from a reversible long-term method that has little or no impact on her blood pressure. Copper IUDs contain no hormones and can be used for up to 12 years.

Estrogen causes fluid and water retention and may be unsuitable for clients with hypertension. Estrogen is contained in COCPs, which are therefore unsuitable for this client. Option B is incorrect because low-dose pills also contain estrogen. Option C is incorrect because bilateral tubal ligation is a permanent contraceptive method, and there is no indication that this client desires a permanent family planning method.

53. (D) Increased libido.

Hyperprolactinemia is an endocrine disorder characterized by an excess secretion of prolactin. It affects both men and women. Symptoms include but are not limited to galactorrhea, infertility, erectile dysfunction, low libido and menstrual irregularities. It can also present as headaches and blurry vision when excess prolactin is secreted by a pituitary tumor.

54. (C) Wear nylon underwear.

Risk factors for urinary tract infections in females include but are not limited to frequent douching, wearing tight underwear made with non-breathable material, poor wiping hygiene, sexual intercourse and urinary tract obstruction. Unlike cotton, nylon is a non-breathable fabric.

55. (C) Stony dull percussion notes on the left anterior chest wall.

Pleural effusion is clinically demonstrated by stony dull percussion notes on the affected side.

56. (B) Dull percussion notes on the right anterior chest wall.

The clinical signs of pneumonia include dull percussion notes, reduced chest wall movement and decreased breath sounds on the affected side.

57. (A) Presence of bubbles when the free end of the tube is placed in water.

The correct location of a nasogastric tube is the esophagus and not the trachea. Immediate signs of improper intubation include choking, coughing and fast breathing. These symptoms may not be prominent in an unconscious patient. Option B is incorrect because the aspiration of a bilious green fluid means the tube is in the stomach. Option C is incorrect because vesicular breath sounds are normal breath sounds. Option D is incorrect because stony dull percussion is a clinical sign of pleural effusion.

58. (A) Inflammation.

Pneumonia is an inflammation of the lung parenchyma. Causes include infectious microbes; toxins like nicotine, carbon and other gases found in cigarettes; and non-biodegradable substances like asbestos, mineral dust and others.

59. (D) Increased mucociliary action.

Asthma is a hyperactive airway disease characterized by bronchiolar hypertrophy, spasms, narrowed airway, increased mucus production and decreased mucociliary activity.

60. (C) Barrel-shaped chest.

The term "blue bloater" is used to describe a client with chronic bronchitis. Chronic bronchitis is a disease of the airway. The bronchioles become infected and inflamed, producing large amounts of mucus. The client attempts to expel this mucus by coughing constantly. Over time, the client develops cyanosis due to decreased oxygen perfusion. Features of chronic bronchitis include chronic productive cough, cyanosis, obesity, pedal edema, fast breathing and chest pain.

61. (B) Chronic productive cough.

The term "pink puffer" is used to describe a client with emphysema. Emphysema is a disease of the air sacs. It is a chronic inflammation of the alveoli. When the alveoli are destroyed, oxygen and carbon dioxide exchange becomes difficult. Also, the lungs gradually lose elasticity and become hyperinflated. Features of emphysema include a barrel-shaped chest, weight loss, fast breathing and chest pain.

62. (B) Diabetic ketoacidosis.

Respiratory acidosis occurs when ineffective respiration causes a buildup of hydrogen ions in the blood. All the options listed are likely causes of respiratory acidosis except diabetic ketoacidosis, which is a cause of metabolic acidosis.

In diabetic ketoacidosis, there is increased production of ketoacids. These acids bind to bicarbonate ions and further worsen the acidotic state.

63. (D) Pott's disease.

Pott's disease is an extrapulmonary manifestation of tuberculosis. It is a chronic degenerative disease of the spine characterized by osteoarthritis and increasing stiffness. Most affected sites of the spine are the upper thoracic and lower lumbar areas.

64. (B) Fluid retention is not in the vascular space.

Nephrotic syndrome is characterized by a loss of proteins and a reduction in plasma oncotic pressure and hydrostatic pressures. These cause a movement of fluid from the intravascular space to the interstitial space. Generalized body edema is a feature of nephrotic syndrome.

65. (C) Blood bags.

The black waste container is used to dispose of cytotoxic drugs, expired drugs, radioactive substances and other non-infectious non-biodegradable materials. Option C is false because infectious plastic materials like blood bags are disposed of in the red waste container.

66. (A) Cap used needles before disposal.

Used needles shouldn't be capped before disposal. This is done to reduce the risk of needle-prick injuries.

67. (C) Sleeping in the same bed.

Scabies is transmitted through prolonged and direct skin contact. It is also transmitted indirectly through fomites like clothes, underwear, towels and bedsheets. Option A is incorrect because scabies is not waterborne. Option B is incorrect because scabies is not an airborne disease.

68. (D) Breastfeed baby for at least two years.

Solid foods are initiated from six months when the baby's stomach is large enough to handle heavy food and the colon has enough flora to digest complex food. Option B is incorrect because babies are breastfed exclusively for six months. Option C is incorrect because infants are not given cow's milk until they are more than a year and a half old.

69. (C) Add a barrier contraceptive to prevent STI transmission.

Option A is incorrect because progesterone-only contraceptives do not reduce the risk of cervical cancers. Option B is incorrect because COCP has a high non-compliance rate. Option D is incorrect because a copper IUD is contraindicated for clients with multiple sexual partners.

70. (A) Calcium chloride.

Calcium chloride or calcium gluconate is given to reduce the risk of ventricular fibrillation. Options B and C are incorrect because salbutamol and insulin are used to drive potassium into the cells. Option D is incorrect because Hartmann's solution is a potassium-containing fluid and therefore is contraindicated in this client.

71. (D) Use of insulin only.

This client has gestational diabetes. She should be started on insulin to reduce the incidence of congenital anomalies, stillbirths, macrosomia, cervical dystocia and other fetal and maternal complications. Oral antidiabetic drugs like metformin are contraindicated in pregnancy.

72. (D) Inquiries should be made about similar symptoms in colleagues and coworkers.

Option A is incorrect because laboratory tests are not usually specific for making a diagnosis. Option B is incorrect because it may not always be necessary or feasible to relocate employees from their work environment before commencing treatment. Option C is incorrect because exposures to hazards that are below the stipulated hazard limit don't rule out the possibility of an occupational health disease.

Many occupational diseases do not cause specific pathognomonic changes in target organ function. A good occupational history is useful in achieving a diagnosis.

73. (C) Physical hazard – sexual harassment at work.

Sexual harassment is a form of psychological hazard. Psychological hazards have negative effects on a worker's mental well-being. Examples include but are not limited to sexual harassment, bias, bullying and victimization.

Physical hazards include environmental factors that are harmful to a worker. Examples include but are not limited to noise, pressure, light, radiation and heights.

74. (C) Serve all food hot.

Foods aren't necessarily served hot, because there are foods that should be served cold, like desserts and salads. The appropriate guideline is to serve hot foods hot and serve cold foods cold.

75. (A) Non-sterile gloves are safe for touching mucous membranes.

Sterile gloves are used to touch mucous membranes and broken skin and for performing sterile procedures. Non-sterile gloves are used for septic procedures and for handling body fluids like blood, urine, semen and saliva. Non-sterile gloves are worn to protect health workers from infection. Sterile gloves work both ways, to protect health workers and clients from cross-contamination.

76. (B) Infected clients should be isolated in negative pressure rooms.

Option A is incorrect because infectious microbes are suspended in the air as particles, aerosols and droplet nuclei. Option C is incorrect because positive pressure rooms are used to isolate immunocompromised clients. Option D is incorrect because disposable N95 masks are used to cover both the nose and mouth.

77. (D) A 25-year-old client with a dislocated ankle.

Compared to the other clients, this client is fairly stable and will be least demanding for the new RN.

78. (C) When the indicator turns on, pierce the pad of the finger.

The side of the finger is pierced. This hurts less.

79. (A) Sodium.

In SIADH, the body secretes excess ADH. This causes the production of concentrated urine. Excess water is retained in the plasma, diluting electrolytes like sodium and causing dilutional hyponatremia.

80. (B) Potassium.

In hypokalemia, ECG changes include flattened and inverted T waves, Q-T interval prolongation, mild ST depression and visible U waves.

81. (D) Assisting clients with feeding.

A nursing assistant can supervise eating, dressing and bathing tasks for a client. A nursing assistant can also assist in measuring vital signs. However, more complex interventions that require clinical reasoning must be done by the RN.

82. (B) Urgency of need.

Nursing interventions are arranged according to the urgency of the client's needs. The goal of every health worker is to keep the client alive and stable.

83. (A) Alert and capacitated.

Before involving clients in their own management, it is important that they are alert and able to understand the medical information given. This should be done before informed consent is obtained. Consent by proxy and durable power of attorney is necessary for clients who are unconscious or incapacitated.

84. (D) They are more proficient in the required knowledge, education and skills.

RNs are more proficient in nursing knowledge, education and skills. As a result, they supervise LPNs and nursing assistants and are responsible for making more complex nursing decisions.

85. (A) A document that contains information about a client's diagnosis and goal of treatment.

Nursing care plans are used to monitor the progress and outcome of a patient. They are created by RNs and are individualized for clients. They are not signed by the American Nurses Association.

86. (C) Treatment.

The nursing process is made up of five sequential processes: assessment, diagnosis, planning, implementation and evaluation.

87. (A) Islam.

Muslims have welcoming rites for a newborn. Part of these rites includes saying a prayer as soon as the baby is born. This prayer is whispered into the right ear of the baby by his father.

88. (B) Shinto.

Shinto is a religion that originates from Japan. Shinto forbids any form of injury to a dead body. It is difficult to obtain consent from Shinto clients for organ donations and autopsies. Option A is incorrect because Jehovah's Witnesses leave donations up to personal choice as long as the organs are drained of blood. Option C is incorrect because Judaism believes organ donation is life-saving. Option D is incorrect because Presbyterians encourage and support organ donation.

89. (A) Hot tea.

The Chinese believe that most illnesses are caused by an imbalance of yin and yang. Yang disorders are cold disorders such as pallor, hypotension and low libido and are treated with hot foods that counterbalance the cold. Yin disorders are hot disorders like fever and are treated with cold foods like iced tea.

90. (D) Hinduism.

Hinduism mandates cremation for dead loved ones. Hindus believe that the dead body is presented as an offering to the god of fire. This offering enables the soul to pass on to the afterlife.

Islam and Judaism forbid cremation. And although Christianity doesn't have a strong opposition to cremation, burial is the preferred form of disposing of a dead body.

91. (D) Probing.

Probing is a barrier to therapeutic communication. In this technique, questions are asked to delve deeper into the client's life. This technique is uncomfortable, and clients may perceive it as a threat to their confidentiality.

92. (C) Ethnographic research.

Quantitative research uses structured methods to obtain numerical data. The aim of quantitative research is to confirm hypotheses about phenomena. This involves quantifying variations between data, predicting causal relationships between data and describing the characteristics of a population. The four main types of quantitative research include the descriptive model, the correlational model, the experimental model and the quasi-experimental model.

93. (D) Surveys.

Primary sources for data include direct sources or firsthand evidence about an event. Examples include audio and video recordings, statistical data, eyewitness accounts and surveys.

94. (A) Video and audio recordings.

Secondary sources of data include data that is collected by someone other than the user. Examples of these data include censuses, surveys and forms of data collected through quantitative and qualitative research methods, i.e., book reviews, surveys, journals, newspaper clippings and so on.

95. (D) It is conducted with a scientific approach to assess quantitative data.

Option A is incorrect because experimental research is a form of quantitative research. Option B is incorrect because this research design isn't an observational study. Option C is incorrect because this research uses close-ended questions.

96. (C) Abstract.

A hypothesis is a statement that assumes a relationship between two variables. It is not abstract but is measurable and tangible.

97. (A) Pedal edema.

Pedal edema is not a specific symptom of preeclampsia. Pedal edema can be a physiological response to reduced blood circulation because of the compression of the IVC by the gravid uterus.

98. (A) Bradycardia.

In the acute phase of hemorrhage, the cardiovascular system attempts to compensate for the blood loss by increasing cardiac activity. Increased heart rate, increased respiratory rate and elevated or normal blood pressure are common signs.

99. (D) Resuscitate with isotonic fluids.

Immediate resuscitation with isotonic fluids is the primary goal. Later, blood may be transfused after assessing the patient's hematocrit. A cervical examination is discouraged during an active bleed because it can worsen bleeding.

100. (D) Gravida 3 para 4.

Gravidity is the sum total of pregnancies, regardless of the outcome. Parity is a measure of viable pregnancies, regardless of the outcome.

Answers to Test 4

1. (B) Independent variable.

An independent variable is a condition that can be changed in an experiment. It is the variable you can control. It is also called a controlled variable.

2. (A) Dependent variable.

A dependent variable is a condition that can be measured in an experiment. It is also called the responding variable.

3. (A) It is task-oriented.

The functional nursing model is designed to encourage efficacy by getting more tasks done in a short period. Several nurses are given specific tasks in the client's management. This model doesn't encourage a client-nurse relationship and it is not client-centered.

4. (A) Tall structure.

A decentralized organization has a flat structure, with feedback going in all directions, including from the bottom up. This organizational structure encourages delegation and autonomy of its members.

5. (C) Charismatic.

Charismatic leaders use communication, motivation and force of personality to inspire their team members to get things done. Charismatic leaders use inspiration, vision, purpose and even spiritual principles to connect to their followers on a deeply emotional level.

6. (D) Autonomy.

Centralized organizations use the top-to-bottom model of communication. They are hierarchical because decisions are made by top executive leaders.

The workers do not have autonomy as they all rely on the leaders and executives to make decisions on behalf of the team.

7. (C) Visionary.

A visionary leader sees the potential of the organization and uses this potential as a tool to encourage team members. Visionary leaders encourage their team members to dream and visualize. They are usually very open to trying new methods that can take the team closer to achieving its potential.

8. (D) Matrix.

The matrix organizational structure is a combination of two or more types of organizational structures. In this structure, there are two chains of command. Employees have dual supervisors, managers and leaders.

9. (A) Decentralized.

In decentralized structures, information flows in all directions without bureaucracy and hindrance. The team members also have independence and autonomy.

10. (D) Studying outcomes on a variable.

Qualitative research isn't used to quantify outcomes because it doesn't analyze numerical data.

11. (A) Qualitative research is used for textual data, while quantitative research is used for numerical data.

Option B is incorrect because qualitative data is used to explore phenomena, while quantitative research is used to form a hypothesis for phenomena. Option C is incorrect because qualitative data has a flexible design, while quantitative research has a stable design. Option D is incorrect because quantitative data uses highly structured formats, while qualitative research uses semi-structured and unstructured techniques.

12. (B) Tofu salad with basmati rice.

Most Hindus avoid eating meat. They believe that eating meat is a violation of other life forms. All other answer options contain meat and are therefore unsuitable.

13. (B) A 49-year-old African American.

The prevalence of hypertension in African Americans is among the highest in the world. Japanese Americans are least likely to develop hypertension due to their diet and body mass.

14. (B) What do you think about making aerobic exercise part of your weekly routine?

Open-ended questions are phrased as statements and require responses that go beyond yes or no. These questions prompt the speaker to talk further and make more information available to the listener.

15. (C) I'm listening.

General lead is a therapeutic communication technique used to inform the speaker that the listener is engaged and attentive to what is being said. It is also used to encourage the speaker to talk further.

16. (B) Giving recognition.

Option A is incorrect because it involves the recognition of nonverbal forms of communication like facial expressions and demeanor. Option C is incorrect because it involves summarizing the emotional content of a speaker's words. Option D is incorrect because it is a non-therapeutic communication technique that is used when the listener thinks the speaker's worries and fears are invalid.

17. (D) Giving advice.

This technique is non-therapeutic because it is evaluative and judgmental. The speaker may feel threatened and refuse to communicate further.

18. (D) I see you don't trust people easily.

This option employs the use of paraphrasing, a therapeutic communication technique that reflects an understanding of the emotional content of the speaker's words. Options A, B and C are incorrect because they use the non-therapeutic techniques of giving advice, presenting reality and probing, respectively.

19. (D) I see you are afraid of vaccines.

This option uses paraphrasing, a therapeutic technique that reflects an understanding of the emotional content of the speaker's words.

Options A, B and C are incorrect because they use the non-therapeutic techniques of evaluating (A, B) and presenting reality (C).

20. (B) Common law.

Common law includes judicial decisions that are made on individual legal cases. They include informed consent, the right to refuse treatment and malpractice.

21. (C) A durable power of attorney.

A durable power of attorney is a written authorization that allows a principal or a guarantor to act on another's behalf.

22. (B) It is not used for illiterate clients.

Informed consent is received from both literate and illiterate clients. The risks and benefits of medical treatment should be communicated to illiterate clients in a way they can understand. All clients should be able to prove that they understand the significance of what was explained to them.

23. (C) Informed consent.

An advance directive is a legal document that describes a client's decisions and preferences for medical treatment when he/she is unable to make and voice these decisions for him/herself. They include a living will, DNR orders, durable power of attorney and a physician order for life-sustaining treatment.

24. (B) It is used to meet specific client goals.

Option A is incorrect because nursing interventions aren't written by physicians but by RNs. Option C is incorrect because dependent interventions require a physician's order. Option D is incorrect because independent interventions are created by RNs.

25. (C) Blood clots.

Blood clots and vaginal bleeding are symptoms of antepartum hemorrhaging. Antepartum hemorrhaging is an emergency condition that is life-threatening to both the mother and the fetus.

26. (B) Administering uterotonics to increase contractions.

The active management of the third stage of labor includes methods used to ensure delivery of the placenta, stimulate uterine contraction and reduce postpartum hemorrhaging. These components include the use of uterotonics to increase contractions, use of controlled cord traction to deliver the placenta and rubbing of the fundus of the uterus to stimulate contraction.

27. (C) Endotracheal tubes with a subglottic port can prevent micro-aspiration.

Option A is incorrect because oral intubation has a lesser risk of transmitting infections than nasal intubation and should be used unless contraindicated. Option B is incorrect because daily oral care with chlorhexidine is indicated for both nasal and oral intubations. Option D is incorrect because endotracheal tubes with bevel ends have no function in reducing nosocomial VAP.

28. (D) Change administration sets and add-in devices daily.

Option A is incorrect because the veins of the upper limb are preferred to the femoral vein. Option B is incorrect because peripheral lines are kept for at least 48 hours to reduce the risk of bloodborne infections. Option C is incorrect because injection ports are cleaned with hypertonic solutions like chlorhexidine.

29. (B) Maintain unobstructed urine flow by hanging the urine bag above the level of the bladder.

The urine bag is kept below the level of the bladder to prevent the backflow of urine and a subsequent UTI.

30. (D) Isolation facilities should have both positive and negative pressure rooms.

Isolation rooms should include negative pressure rooms for those who are infectious and positive pressure rooms for those who need protective isolation. Option A is incorrect because hospital-acquired microbes are virulent and survive for a long time in certain environments. Option B is incorrect because the ICU should be located away from the main wards. Option C is incorrect because the space between beds should be at least 3.5 cm.

31. (D) Systemic intravenous antibiotics are indicated for a short time.

Systemic antibiotics are used for a short time before switching to topical antibiotics.

Option A is incorrect because plants and flowers are potential sources of infection and are therefore not allowed into burn centers. Option B is incorrect because human tetanus immunoglobulin is given to all clients regardless of their immunization status. Option C is incorrect because topical antibiotics are applied to the dressing then applied to the burn site.

32. (B) The most important safety precaution is handwashing.

Option A is incorrect because transplant clients are immunosuppressed and should be kept in protective isolation rooms with positive pressure. Option C is incorrect because antibiotics are not given as prophylaxis unless indicated. Option D is incorrect because live-attenuated vaccines are contraindicated for clients with severe immunosuppression.

33. (A) The cord will fall off in two to four weeks.

The cord falls off in 7–10 days. An umbilical cord that lasts more than two weeks is abnormal. In such cases, the mother should consult a pediatrician.

34. (C) Commence prophylactic folic acid supplementation from 16 weeks of gestation.

Folic acid is needed for the formation of the neural tube in fetuses. This process is completed by the fourth week of conception. Folic acid should be commenced as soon as the mother thinks she is pregnant. Ideally, folic acid supplementation is necessary for every woman who wishes to become pregnant. It is used as part of preconception care.

35. (D) Health-care workers with weeping infections of the hands shouldn't be excluded from direct contact with patients, as long as they wear sterile gloves.

Health workers with weeping hand infections should be excluded from offering direct care to patients.

36. (B) Progesterone and estradiol are assayed on day 21.

Option A is incorrect because FSH, LH and estradiol are assayed on day 3. Option C is incorrect because a high FSH level is indicative of poor ovarian reserve and possible infertility. Option D is incorrect because LH and FSH are released by the pituitary gland, while estradiol is released by the ovaries. Progesterone and estradiol are assayed on day 21. A low progesterone level is indicative of an anovulatory cycle.

37. (D) Bladder irrigation.

Acute nephritic syndrome is a disease of the kidneys characterized by hematuria, hypertension and azotemia. Management principles include control of blood pressure, fluid intake and restricted protein and salt intake. Bladder irrigation is not useful because hematuria is a result of damage to the kidneys' nephrons, and not the bladder.

38. (D) Polyhydramnios.

Potter's syndrome is a spectrum of congenital renal defects used to characterize fetuses born with genetic diseases of the kidneys. These neonates also have oligohydramnios, pulmonary hypoplasia and deformities of the limbs such as clubbed feet. Genetic disorders of the kidney include polycystic kidney disease, bilateral renal agenesis and post-urethral valve.

39. (D) An elderly patient with urinary incontinence.

Urinary incontinence is characterized by involuntary voiding of urine. Posterior urethral valve is a common cause of urinary tract infections in males. It is an obstructive uropathy characterized by poor urine flow and hydronephrosis. The retention of urine and backflow of urine predisposes clients to chronic urinary tract infections. Candidiasis is also a common cause of urinary tract infections; a client with a neurogenic bladder can be incontinent or suffer from chronic obstruction. However, chronic urinary tract infections are a complication for a client with a neurogenic bladder.

40. (A) Urine volume.

The nephron is the functional unit of the kidneys. It is responsible for the filtration and absorption of water and solutes. Impaired urinary function is characterized by poor urinary filtration and water reabsorption.

41. (A) Posterior urethral valve.

Posterior urethral valve is a post-renal (obstructive) cause of kidney disease. Renal causes of kidney disease involve pathological processes that occur primarily in the kidneys. Examples include genetic malformation of the kidneys, kidney infections, nephritic and nephrotic diseases, tumors and others.

42. (A) Aspirin is given for chronic groin pain.

Like other NSAIDs, the use of aspirin is contraindicated in chronic kidney disease. NSAIDs and aminoglycosides are potential nephrotoxins that worsen urinary function.

43. (C) Porphyria.

Although clients with porphyria present with urine that becomes increasingly reddish on oxidation, porphyria is not a cause of hematuria. Porphyrins accumulate in the blood, affecting the skin and nervous system. Symptoms include abdominal pain, vomiting, constipation, fever, high blood pressure and tachycardia.

44. (C) Control temperature.

A febrile convulsion is a possible complication in this child with a high-grade fever. Such febrile convulsions are either complex or simple generalized tonic-clonic seizures lasting less than fifteen minutes. Pain relief, antibiotics and fluids can be commenced after controlling the client's temperature.

45. (D) Orthopnea.

Right-sided heart failure is an inability of the right ventricles to pump blood into the lungs. As a result, blood backs up in the venous circulation, causing pedal edema, ascites and congestion of the liver and spleen. Option D is incorrect because orthopnea is a feature of left-sided heart failure.

46. (C) Pedal edema.

Left-sided heart failure occurs when the left ventricles are unable to pump oxygenated blood into the systemic circulation. As a result, blood congests the lungs. Pulmonary edema causes fast breathing, orthopnea and paroxysmal nocturnal tachypnea. Pedal edema is a feature of right-sided heart failure.

47. (B) Prompt cardiac compressions.

A client with these symptoms likely has pulmonary edema or a pulmonary embolism. Supplemental oxygen is needed to improve oxygen saturation. Intravenous diuretics like Lasix are useful if there is pulmonary edema. Fibrinolytics are useful to lyse circulating clots. Cardiac compressions have no role in improving oxygen saturation in this client.

48. (D) It can be treated with Calcitonin.

Option A is incorrect because hypercalcemia occurs when serum calcium is greater than 2.6 mmol/L. Option B is incorrect because tetanic seizures are complications of hypocalcemia. Symptoms of hypercalcemia include but are not limited to abdominal pain, nausea, vomiting, constipation, the formation of kidney stones and arrhythmia. Option C is incorrect because hyperthyroidism is a cause of hypercalcemia.

49. (D) Tetany.

Symptoms of hyperkalemia include but are not limited to numbness, tingling sensation in the hands and feet, chest pain, palpitations, arrhythmia, nausea and vomiting. Tetany is a clinical sign of hypocalcemia.

50. (A) Early ambulation.

Obesity is a risk factor for deep vein thrombosis and pulmonary embolisms. Reduced blood circulation and blood stasis are likely to cause a thrombotic state in the deep veins. Early ambulation is necessary to improve blood circulation.

Option B is indicated for clients with pedal edema and deep venous thrombosis. Option C is indicated for clients with anorexia. Option D is indicated for bedridden clients.

51. (C) Ventricular septal defect.

In cyanotic congenital heart diseases, deoxygenated blood bypasses the lungs and enters the systemic circulation. It is caused by structural defects of the heart that cause right-to-left shunting and increase pulmonary vascular resistance.

52. (A) 3:1.

The compression to ventilation ratio is 3:1. A minute's resuscitation includes 90 compressions to 30 breaths. Higher ratios can be used if the apnea is of cardiac origin, i.e., 15:2.

53. (C) Squatting temporarily reverses the right-to-left shunt.

Children with tetralogy of Fallot develop Tet spells. Tet spells are also called hypercyanotic spells. They are a sudden exacerbation of cyanosis that occurs when the patient is agitated, crying or eating. Symptoms include breathlessness, cyanosis, anxiety and syncope. Older children squat to get relief. This is because squatting increases systemic vascular resistance and temporarily reverses the right-to-left shunting of deoxygenated blood.

54. (C) A 23-year-old male client with a urethral stricture and acute urinary retention.

Acute urinary obstruction is an indication for urethral catheterization. The client with Parkinson's can benefit from adult diapers. The client with chronic leg ulcers is ambulatory and doesn't need to be catheterized. The client with right-sided heart failure needs an adult diaper or a bedpan. Urinary tract infections are a complication of prolonged urethral catheterization; therefore, urethral catheters should be used only as a last resort.

55. (C) A two-month-old female with breathlessness caused by acute heart failure.

This child is at risk of aspiration. Also, if she doesn't eat properly, she is at risk of malnutrition. The other patients have no risk of aspiration, and diverse methods can be employed to encourage feeding. The immunosuppressed client should be treated with oral nystatin, and the chemotherapy client should be encouraged to eat small, frequent meals.

56. (B) This client is underweight.

Option A is incorrect because a body mass index that is less than 18.5 kg/m^2 is underweight. Option C is incorrect because cachexia is measured by assessment of skin thickness, prominence of facial bones and the presence of loose skin folds.

Option D is incorrect because malnourishment is diagnosed by assessing the client's nutritional and diet history and other biophysical factors apart from weight.

57. (A) A fast respiratory rate.

The normal respiratory rate in a two-year-old child is within 40–50 cycles per minute. Option D is incorrect because bronchial breath sounds are assessed during auscultation and not during an inspection.

58. (C) A normal heart rate.

The heart rate of a two-year-old is expected to be 100–120 bpm. Option D is incorrect because heart sounds are assessed during auscultation and not during an inspection.

59. (D) A client with aphasia.

This client is not at risk for aspiration because aphasia is not a disorder of the pharynx but of the speech centers in the brain.

The risk for aspiration occurs when there is impairment of the higher center, as seen in unconsciousness. Aspiration can also occur in a nervous impairment of the gag reflex and in an impairment of the upper and lower esophageal sphincters.

60. (D) Mallory–Weiss syndrome.

Mallory–Weiss syndrome is described as bleeding from lacerations in the muscles of the gastroesophageal junction. It is caused by retching and excessive vomiting.

Complications of chronic constipation include anal fissures, fecal impaction and fecal incontinence.

61. (B) The client is at risk for diabetic ketoacidosis.

HbA1c of more than 6.2% is diagnostic of poor diabetic control. This client needs to be counseled on the correlation between optimal glycemic control and reduced risks for acute and chronic complications of diabetes. Option C is incorrect because the client is at risk of hyperglycemic emergencies. Option D is incorrect because the client has diabetes mellitus and not impaired glucose tolerance.

62. (A) A vaginal examination to assess the cause of bleeding.

A vaginal examination is contraindicated in this patient because there is a risk of worsening the bleeding if she has a placenta previa. An obstetric ultrasound scan should be done to assess placentation before a vaginal examination is performed.

63. (A) Metabolic alkalosis.

This client has excess bicarbonate ions. In severe vomiting, there is a loss of hydrogen and chloride ions in the vomitus. As a result, there is a net shift of bicarbonate ions into the extracellular space.

64. (C) Respiratory acidosis.

This client is hypercapnic because there is an accumulation of carbon dioxide in the bloodstream. In asthma, there is constriction and hypertrophy of the bronchioles. This action impairs inspiration and gaseous exchange of oxygen for carbon dioxide. As a result of this, carbon dioxide builds up in the blood, causing hypercapnia.

65. (D) Tuberculin bacilli.

Anaphylaxis is an immediate hypersensitivity reaction (Type 1) mediated by IgE antibodies. Causes are numerous and include common allergens in food, drugs (including NSAIDs and beta-lactam antibiotics) and venom from insect bites. Less common causes include latex and semen. Tuberculin bacilli cause a delayed T-cell-mediated hypersensitivity reaction (Type 4). This reaction is found in many chronic infectious diseases like tuberculosis and fungus. It is also the immune response to BCG vaccines.

66. (A) Acknowledge the client's perception of pain.

The client's perception of pain must be acknowledged as valid. Pain is measured using standardized pain scales. The collected data is acknowledged, and then treatment modalities are implemented based on the results from the data.

67. (C) A urine output of 15 ml/hr.

Signs and symptoms of magnesium sulfate toxicity include an absence of deep tendon reflexes, hypotension, respiratory depression and low urine output.

68. (D) Vitamin A.

Vitamin A, also known as retinoic acid, is contraindicated during pregnancy. It is teratogenic and implicated in first trimester miscarriages and congenital malformations of the cardiac and nervous systems. Fersolate, folic acid and vitamin C are required for heme synthesis. Folic acid is required for the healthy formation of the nervous system.

69. (B) May complain of a cough.

Option A is incorrect because a routine investigation of potassium is required to detect hyperkalemia. Option C is incorrect because ACE inhibitors are contraindicated in pregnancy. Option D is incorrect because ACE inhibitors are potassium-sparing antihypertensives.

70. (D) Fresh whole blood.

Since the child is in hemorrhagic shock, he will benefit from both the red blood cells and clotting factors contained in fresh whole blood. Platelet concentrate is not indicated because the clotting disorder is not from a lack of platelets but from a lack of clotting factors.

71. (C) They reduce bone growth and density.

Although corticosteroids cause the other effects listed above, special attention must be taken when prescribing these to children because they increase the resorption of calcium from the bones and stimulate early closure of growth plates in long bones. These actions reduce bone growth and bone density.

72. (C) It can cause tinnitus.

Tinnitus or ringing in the ears is caused by an overdose of acetylsalicylic acid. Option A is incorrect because gastric ulcers are a complication of acetylsalicylic acid, and therefore it shouldn't be taken on an empty stomach. Option B is incorrect because antacids impair the absorption of acetylsalicylic acid. Option D is incorrect because although acetylsalicylic acid reduces the risk of myocardial infarction, it is no use in controlling hypertension.

73. (B) It's also known as the scientific name.

A chemical name is a scientific name. These are typically very long and too complex to be used in conversational speech. Generic/proprietary names are different from the chemical name.

74. (B) Generic name.

Rosuvastatin is a generic name for a group of statin drugs used to reduce cholesterol levels. These statin drugs are the first-line drugs used in the treatment of dyslipidemia and atherosclerosis. The brand names of rosuvastatin include Rosastin, Colcardiol, Colfri, Crestor, Crativ and Diliva. The popular brand name Lipitor is for the generic statin drug, atorvastatin.

75. (B) The trade name is sildenafil.

Viagra is Pfizer's brand name for sildenafil. It is used to treat erectile dysfunction in males, Reynaud's phenomenon and pulmonary hypertension. Common side effects include hypotension, dizziness, flushed skin and headaches.

76. (C) Potentiation.

Potentiation describes a drug action when a drug is given to increase the action of another drug. Agonists are drugs that bind to a receptor to stimulate a biological response.

77. (D) A combination of allopurinol and methotrexate.

Synergism is used to describe a drug action where two drugs act together to improve a therapeutic outcome. Penicillin is used with an aminoglycoside to treat bacterial infections. Penicillin damages the cell wall of a gram-positive bacteria, allowing the penetration of gentamycin. Aspirin and caffeine are combined to increase the analgesic effect. Probenecid and penicillin are combined because probenecid slows down the excretion of penicillin.

78. (C) Streptomycin.

The first-line anti-Koch's drugs are rifampicin, isoniazid, pyrazinamide and ethambutol.

79. (B) Ethambutol.

The side effects of ethambutol include optic neuritis characterized by reduced visual acuity and color blindness.

80. (C) Lindane.

Both children will benefit from all the drugs mentioned in the answer choices except lindane. Although lindane is indicated in treating scabies, its use is contraindicated in children less than two years old because of its neurotoxic effect.

81. (C) Caffeine.

Neonates with small-sized VSDs can be given NSAIDs to hasten the closure of the VSD. Caffeine is not an NSAID.

82. (C) Lomotil.

Lomotil is an antimotility drug that is used to treat diarrhea. The other drugs are all used to improve intestinal motility. Dulcolax is a suppository. Milk of magnesia is an osmotic laxative, while bisacodyl is an intestinal irritant.

83. (C) A client with macular degeneration in both eyes.

A white cane is used for the visually impaired client. The cane is longer, thinner and ideal for proprioception. The cane is also used to alert motorists and pedestrians that the user is visually impaired.

84. (A) Empty colostomy pouch only when it is completely full.

To prevent leaks and odors, a colostomy pouch is emptied when it is one-third or half full.

85. (B) Prolapse – a part of the bowel pushes out of the stoma.

Stenosis is a narrowing of the stoma. A hernia occurs when a part of the bowel pushes around the area of the stoma. Retraction occurs when the stoma sinks below the skin level.

86. (C) Do a clean catch.

A urine sample from a two-month-old male is collected by a clean catch, either from anticipating the child's next urination or tying a sterile plastic bag around the tip of the phallus. Catheterization is painful and uncomfortable and has a risk of causing a urinary tract infection. Urine obtained from a diaper is contaminated and unsuitable.

87. (B) Suctioning every two hours.

Suctioning is done based on a clinical indication. Too-frequent suctioning can cause hypoxia.

88. (D) Restricting fluid intake to prevent congestive cardiac failure.

A client with fever is at risk of dehydration. The client should be encouraged to drink fluids liberally to keep hydrated.

89. (D) Serve food hot to prevent spasms.

The client should avoid eating too-hot or too-cold foods to prevent coughs and spasms.

90. (B) Psychological.

In psychological dependence, a client can't stop using a substance because of the feeling he derives from using the drug. Psychological dependence is commonly seen in opioids, nicotine and cannabis use.

91. (D) Examine your feelings and beliefs about suicide.

As a nurse offering professional health services to a suicidal client, you should take the time to reflect and examine your feelings towards suicide. This examination will reduce the risks of displaying bias and prejudice in your nursing care.

92. (C) Provide a safe environment with good security.

Although all the answer options are necessary, it is important to first make sure that the client is in a safe environment. Memory loss and personality changes increase the danger to this client's safety.

93. (B) Sudden onset.

Delirium and dementia may present with similar symptoms, but a distinguishing characteristic is the onset of these symptoms. Dementia has an insidious onset, while delirium is sudden in onset.

94. (A) Episodic binge eating and induced vomiting.

Options B and C are incorrect because anorexia and bulimia are both eating disorders with associated low self-esteem and body dysmorphia. Option D is incorrect because anorexic patients are underweight with reduced body mass indexes. Unlike bulimia, anorexics don't binge eat but starve themselves.

95. (B) Voluntary.

Malingering is a conscious production of false or exaggerated physical or psychological symptoms with the aim of a reward. Both malingering and somatoform disorders are psychological and physical, and both are done for a reward. However, malingering is voluntary, while somatoform disorders are unconscious.

96. (D) Tennis.

All the other activities have a high risk for anorexia because they put an emphasis on low body fat and aesthetics.

97. (B) Dull.

A healthy liver is dull on percussion. A liver is a solid organ located in the right hypochondrium region. In cirrhosis, the liver is fibrosed and has healthy liver tissues that are interspersed in fibrous tissue. As a result, a cirrhotic liver can be tympanic on percussion.

98. (C) A ventricular dilation.

The apex beat is usually heard at the fifth left intercostal space (LICS), midclavicular line (MCL). A displaced apex beat can be seen in ventricular hypertrophy such as in hypertensive heart diseases or hypertrophic cardiomyopathy and also in dilated cardiomyopathy.

99. (D) Corneal reflex – Cranial nerve III.

The corneal reflex is mediated by the ophthalmic branch of the trigeminal nerve (Cranial nerve V).

100. (D) A premature two-week-old male with a PDA.

Finger clubbing is caused by a variety of diseases that stimulate the release of growth factors from the blood cells. These blood cells lodge in the nail-bed capillary and stimulate the growth of vascular connective tissue. Causes of finger clubbing include cyanotic congenital heart diseases, infective endocarditis, lung diseases, liver diseases and inflammatory bowel diseases.

Made in the USA
Middletown, DE
06 November 2020

23427795R00230